SKINNY REVISITED:
Rethinking Anorexia Nervosa and Its Treatment

Maria Baratta

NASW PRESS

National Association of Social Workers
Washington, DC

James J. Kelly, PhD, ACSW, LCSW, President
Elizabeth J. Clark, PhD, ACSW, MPH, Executive Director

Cheryl Y. Bradley, *Publisher*
Lisa M. O'Hearn, *Managing Editor*
John Cassels, *Project Manager and Staff Editor*
Wayson Jones, *Copyeditor*
Rebecca Tippets, *Proofreader*
Tom Fish, *Indexer*

Cover by Eye to Eye Design Studio
Interior design by Electronic Quill
Printed and bound by Victor Graphics

First impression: May 2011

Library of Congress Cataloging-in-Publication Data

Baratta, Maria, 1954–
  Skinny revisited: rethinking anorexia nervosa and its treatment / Maria Baratta.
     p.   cm.
  Includes bibliographical references and index.
  ISBN 978-0-87101-407-8
  1. Anorexia nervosa. 2. Beauty, Personal. I. Title.
  RC522.A5B37 2011
  616.85'262—dc22

                                                                                  2011014047

Printed in the United States of America

Contents

About the Author

Maria Baratta, PhD, LCSW, ACSW, BCD, is a clinical social worker in private practice in New York City. Dr. Baratta has taught social work courses in the Department of Sociology and Anthropology, St. John's University, and published several articles. She has treated patients with eating disorders for over 25 years.

Acknowledgments

This book originated in the form of a scribbled, scotch-taped book that I wrote for fun when I was seven. My parents actually kept that book for many years in hope of inspiring me to write. For their belief in me as an author, their love and support, I am forever grateful. And I will always appreciate and love my mother, Palma, for her unfailing enthusiasm for anything I have ever done, and my father, Joe, for his original insights.

I must also acknowledge the best family ever: my brother Pat, for his friendship and love, and my brother Joe and sister-in-law Donna, with love and gratitude for their presence in my life. To my nieces Dina, Donna, and Danielle and my goddaughter Kristen: May you always realize your beauty and potential. And this book is offered in loving memory to my 100 percent Italian Gramma Maria Baratta—God rest her soul—whom I adored and who cooked the best, *best* everything with unconditional love.

Heartfelt thanks to Steven Daniel of IUGS, for his encouragement and faith in me while I was writing my doctoral dissertation, from which this book was derived, and to Lorenzo Margini, for clinical review and encouraging me in the process. Thanks also to Eric Hollander for his clinical input.

A huge thank you to my editor at NASW Press, John Cassels, for his hard work and heart and for turning my writing into respectable English; enormous gratitude to Lisa M. O'Hearn, managing editor of the Press, for believing in this endeavor from the outset; and special thanks to publisher extraordinaire Cheryl Y. Bradley and the rest of the staff at NASW Press for their impressive talent.

I am deeply grateful to my wonderful patients throughout the years who inspired what I have written.

Thank you to the following friends: Kathy Maffucci, Christine Jiminez, Anthony Morris, Kitty Dunne, Michelle Pinto, and Rosanne DiBiase.

Finally, words cannot express how much I appreciate and adore brilliant, wonderful Matthew, for endless patience with my frantic cries for tech support, for the laughs we shared over my questionable English, for editing, for having faith in me, and for being the best, most amazing son ever. I love you tons. And to God, for this blessing, thank you.

To Matthew

Introduction

Women are rarely satisfied with the way they look. There is always something wrong or something they don't like about their appearance. Why is it that women are known to walk into a room and do a "once over" to assess themselves in comparison with the other women in the room and subsequently adjust how they "feel" on the basis of how they measure up in terms of looks? And depending how we feel or who we compare ourselves to, we can feel either "thin" or "fat," having nothing to do with body size or weight. Women know what I mean. Why is it that women seldom eat what they really want? There are always self-imposed limits to what and how much they eat in order to look "good" and fit into something trendy. And something trendy is *always* small. We are never okay just the way we are. We have "bad hair days," we have "nothing to wear," our shoes hurt and we "feel fat." We are constantly surrounded by something or some way to improve ourselves—something we can buy, a product with a promise, or something we can do, be it a diet, a procedure, or surgery. The quest for beauty is endless.

Our cultural preoccupation with thinness is unavoidable. We are surrounded by images of skinny women—magazines, billboards, television— questionably airbrushed images. For women, self-esteem and appearance are intertwined and based on a culturally predetermined ideal body— hardly realistic when each person's body is different. It certainly makes logical sense that women engage in disordered eating as a means of achieving a thin, culturally idealized body. Anorexia nervosa is a psychiatric disorder characterized by a willful determination to control the intake of food to

1

the point of starvation, one that is precipitated by a myriad of causative factors. All too often, anorexia is an ultimate, overwhelming obsession with the ideal of an unequivocally skinny body—and a life-threatening means of achieving it.

Some of us remember where we were the day man first set foot on the moon. I remember what I was eating. For someone who grew up in an Italian family, it's certainly not unusual to remember a meal. What I know to be true is that food is love and celebration and comfort and sustenance; food is everywhere and everything. So I guess it makes perfect antithetical sense for me, as a psychotherapist, to have taken an exceptional interest in anorexia nervosa.

My personal interest in self-imposed starvation began when I was about 12 years old. I had a cousin who visited from time to time who was very skinny and simply refused to eat. But she looked good in the latest fashions, and she didn't have to hold her breath to zip up a skirt. The family was always in an uproar when she visited because she did the unthinkable: She rejected food—really great food. My grandmother would cook for hours; her house had the most heavenly aroma of marinara sauce, detectable three houses away. To me, this made it altogether impossible to even consider not eating, hungry or not. I was fascinated by my cousin's ability to unaffectedly dismiss food. The adults were beyond aggravated and forever worried, always coaxing her to eat, but to no avail. They would say, "Why can't you eat like . . .?"—and they would point to me, and I was confused as to whether it was a compliment or an insult. I remember my aunt's unrelenting warning that if you didn't eat, you would die. She said this hoping that her daughter would take heed. After my cousin left, my family would talk about her for weeks, in dismay and utter disbelief. I wanted to understand.

I grew up in the 1960s and remember when, once a year, you were weighed in front of your entire class. I still cringe when I recall my fifth-grade teacher choosing the cutest boy in the class to call out everyone's weight so that she could write it down. I really don't know why they needed to record everyone's weight, but, one by one, we were called to step on a scale, and our weight was announced for the entire world to hear. As if that wasn't bad enough, a few would have to go the nurse's office. We all knew what that meant, and I always held my breath for a few seconds and prayed not to be sent to the nurse for eating too many of my grandmother's meatballs. Being sent to the nurse meant that you were either underweight or overweight, either of which warranted a note home to your parents. That was worse than a bad report card. And to make matters worse still, those were the infamous days when Twiggy, an emaciated British model who appeared to never have eaten a dish of lasagna, had lowered the bar for weight and thinness in the fashion world and set a standard for body size that few could attain.

It was the beginning of an era in our culture marked by weight obsession and the emergence of the diet industry. Women were burning bras and fighting for equal rights. It was during those years that I became keenly aware of the juxtaposition between the pressure for women to be skinny and the pressure for women to be equal to and competitive with men. There were moments when it seemed as if women really could compete with men and enjoy equal opportunities for career directives. Yet, at the very same time, the fashion industry began to present women with a new ideal body image that was far thinner than ever before. "Skinny," as an ideal, was all over the place, and women's bodies and clothing sizes were shrinking. Women have always been known to read magazines, and these were filled with repetitive and unavoidable images of skinny women. Those were the days when the door opened for the diet industry to flourish and invent bizarre regimens, all aimed at helping women achieve the Twiggy look. As an adolescent girl, I remember feeling the pressure of having to become skinny to fit into a mini skirt like Twiggy and having to diet to do so. But it was confusing—was skinny good or bad?

When man set foot on the moon, I was on an "ice cream diet," eating a bowl of peppermint stick ice cream while on vacation with my family. I had been eating only ice cream for breakfast, lunch, and dinner. My brothers thought it was stupid. My parents didn't try to convince me to abandon it because they knew it wouldn't last. I ate ice cream all over New England, and by the time we returned home, I was hungry and never wanted to eat ice cream again. I eventually made peace with the fact that I was not going to look like Twiggy, no matter how, or how much, I rationed my food. And I was not sure if that was bad or good.

Nevertheless, I was motivated to understand the cultural forces that caused otherwise reasonable women to diet unnecessarily, starving themselves to achieve a certain look. I took issue with the pervasive cultural pressure for women to undermine their bodies' natural, comfortable set-point weight. I wondered why women complained of "feeling fat" and obsessed over being thin—a standard that did not seem to apply to men the way it did to women. Perhaps the current epidemic of obesity in the United States is a swing of the pendulum in the entirely opposite direction—a reaction formation of sorts. Perhaps Americans are giving up and overdoing it because the cultural ideal of "skinny" is so far out of reach for many. Perhaps our current antiobesity climate is an ultimate pronouncement that "skinny" still rules.

This book contains an overview of anorexia nervosa from a feminist sociobehavioral perspective and a treatment model for clinicians. Although the book is intended for clinicians, those close to an anorexic may also benefit by familiarizing themselves with the strategies used in psychotherapeutic treatment—which may, in turn, provide some insight and direction for guiding an anorexic back to health. Through a better understanding of the disorder, those close to an anorexic may approach the patient with a more tolerant and informed attitude, thus supporting and facilitating treatment interventions.

My work is based on 28 years of clinical practice and many successful treatments of anorexic patients. I present a treatment model that has evolved from my deep concern for the phenomenon of women feeling pressured to be "skinny" and starving their bodies to do so. My treatment approach has demonstrated the ability to overcome the willfulness and marked resistance to therapeutic intervention that usually occurs in attempts to treat anorexia. I have managed to address the biggest problem in treating anorexia, which is the marked resistance to any kind of intervention. I have also found a way to give the anorexic patient control over her food intake, control aimed in the direction of healthy weight and recovery.

This book also provides an overview of anorexia nervosa itself, using both theoretical and practice-based perspectives. I present theoretical approaches that are consistent with my work and have informed and influenced my treatment approach. I provide a definition of anorexia nervosa as a composite of the literature and describe symptoms as they are reflected in research. I also provide a narrative description of how anorexia is a feminist issue and how the culture at large has largely contributed to its existence. As part of an overview of the disorder, I explain, from a sociobehavioral perspective, the manifestation of anorexia in a postfeminist era. To support my premise, I include clinical case studies and explain the treatment of anorexia nervosa in theory and from my own clinical perspective.

One day, while in the midst of researching anorexia, I entered a college bookstore, where I found—prominently displayed for young women to see—a book titled *Skinny Bitch: A No-Nonsense, Tough Love Guide for Savvy Girls Who Want to Stop Eating Crap and Start Looking Fabulous!* (Freedman & Barnouvin, 2005). It was upsetting to me that a book promoting the ideology that "looking fabulous" requires being "skinny" was in a university bookstore—especially considering how prevalent eating disorders are among young women! Horrified by the title, I picked up the book and began reading, and what I read validated my contention that women continue to be unnecessarily pressured to value "skinny" and strive for thinness, no matter how aware of the dangers they are. *Skinny Bitch* was published in 2005, when political correctness seemed to have somehow become separated from the subject of women and their relationships with their bodies, evidenced by the book's bearing the "#1 *New York Times* Bestseller" seal on its cover. Women have always had tenuous relationships with their bodies and have always been pressured to meet impossible cultural standards for beauty; the extreme of that pressure is manifest in the prevalence of anorexia nervosa.

Impressionable young women have read and will be reading books that encourage dissatisfaction with their bodies—dissatisfaction that, in turn, feeds into and reinforces a dysfunctional cultural climate that breeds eating disorders. Even worse, and more dangerous, are proanorexia (or "pro-ana") Web sites that promote anorexia and encourage disordered eating as what the site creators deem "a lifestyle choice." Anorexia can lead to death and numerous serious health complications, such as compromised fertility and pregnancy, muscle and bone loss, and heart damage (which notably caused the death of Karen Carpenter), to name just a few (Shaw, 2005). Viewed through a sociological lens, there appears to have been a strong cultural influence, historic in nature, encouraging women to prove their worthiness through self-imposed starvation, and that notion has carried through to the present. There is something terribly wrong with this picture.

According to feminist author Susie Orbach, our culture at large has been the cause of "body hatred" among women of all ages. Orbach (2008) contended that 90 percent of all women want to change one aspect of their appearance, only 2 percent of women are able to refer to themselves as "beautiful," and 70 to 80 percent of women manipulate their eating. In her research, Orbach found that 72 percent of girls and 68 percent of women avoided ordinary activities because they felt "awful" about their looks, and that dieting has a 97 percent failure rate. In the course of a week, women are exposed to about 3,000 images of skinny women—"lollipop" women with extremely skinny bodies and large, disproportionate heads, images of whom appear constantly in advertisements and magazines. Women form relationships with their own bodies on the basis of these images in the media.

Yet women were not always expected to be "skinny." In the American Movie Classics television series *Mad Men,* we are given an opportunity to observe things as they were in the early 1960s, before the Twiggy era. Watching *Mad Men,* we see children playing happily with plastic dry cleaners' bags over their heads, we marvel at widespread smoking, and we can't help but notice that the women of those prefeminist years were curvy—very curvy. But shortly after, as the feminist movement became the voice that challenged women's second-class citizenship, the cultural norm for women's bodies seemed to shrink. Curvy seemed to be replaced with skinny, angular, and boy-like. In *The Beauty Myth,* Naomi Wolf (1991) made the connection between the importance of beauty for women and their attainment of power. There were cultural influences that determined those body ideals—a conspiracy of sorts, aimed at keeping women and their perennial fight for equality with men at bay. Wolf contended that the "beauty myth" was about men's institutions and institutional power waging a counteroffensive against women, aiming to defeat women's strength with the expectation of thinness. At the point in history when women were gaining equality with men, the "skinny" archetype—lank, underfed, and weakened—emerged into cultural prominence. A similar effect occurred during the 1920s' "flapper days," when women finally got the right to vote. Women earned rights, and "skinny" emerged as the new norm. And eating disorders became prevalent.

Anorexia Observed in My Clinical Practice

Early in my practice as a psychotherapist, I began working with anorexics and understood that treating anorexia was a "holy grail" of sorts in the treatment world. It was widely known that those suffering from anorexia nervosa were very difficult, if not impossible, to treat. Yet our universal need to survive as a species makes it imperative that we find a way to lead anorexics back to healthy eating. What later evolved into my treatment approach was originally a careful and respectful challenge of the anorexic's relationship with food through language. Outwardly, anorexics appear to reject food, starving themselves, yet inwardly they are hungry, *literally* hungry—how could they not be? Because there is comorbidity between anorexia and obsessive–compulsive disorder, I found that anorexic patients were amenable to allowing me to obsess about food with them. In fact, if you talk about food enough, you will get hungry. The anorexic's willful refusal to eat is a defense against the longing to eat. My premise was to challenge the willful defense of starvation by appealing to the obsessional nature of the disorder, using logic, and thus replacing unhealthy obsessional eating with obsessing about healthy eating. This is an ideal use of a cognitive–behavioral intervention.

Joan Brumberg (2000) began her book about anorexia, *Fasting Girls: The History of Anorexia Nervosa,* with this statement: "I am not a recovered anorexic nor am I the mother of an anorexic daughter" (p. 3). It is important for me, also, to state that I, too, am neither a recovered anorexic nor the mother of an anorexic daughter. I began my psychotherapy practice in the early 1980s, and as a family psychotherapist, I began to see more than a few Italian American patients worried about daughters who were "too skinny" and refused to eat. And so I began to treat anorexics as an offshoot of my work as a family therapist who treated numerous members of a family from a family systems theoretical approach. For Italians, the "refusal to eat" was a crisis and a cause for concern that prompted the seeking of professional intervention, even though Italians as a cultural group were chronically in denial and self-reliant when it came to mental illness, seldom seeking professional help.

My early work began with treatment of the daughters of my original patients, who had been treated for unrelated psychiatric conditions and had experienced successful treatment outcomes. Some time later, I would be asked to treat the anorexic daughter. "My daughter won't eat, and she's too skinny—that's not normal, and you need to see her" was the phrase with which several of my first anorexic patients were referred. One of my first anorexic patients was the daughter of a patient I was treating for depression; she had initially attended family sessions as part of her mother's treatment. The daughter's bizarre eating rituals slowly began to surface and were discussed in the context of the family sessions. As it became apparent that the daughter was possibly anorexic, I began the assessment and engagement phase of the treatment process.

The first intervention involved tentatively and cautiously interviewing the patient individually to determine if there was a viable treatment situation. I then met with the parents together with the patient and proceeded to meet with the patient individually, including her in family sessions when needed. Consistently, the patient would engage in treatment with marked resistance and refuse all other psychotherapeutic intervention and referrals. Initially, my concern for the patient's self-reported refusal to eat and visibly emaciated state necessitated referral to an eating disorder hospital unit to address the medical crisis and stabilize her weight. After having spent some time in the hospital as an inpatient, however, the patient returned to me still skinny—at the referral of the treating physician, who, at the time, stated to me on the telephone, "She's all yours; she actually wants to see you, and that's better than how she's doing here." There was a willfulness and marked resistance to therapeutic intervention that, for some reason, I was able to overcome. And so began my work with anorexics.

The more I have researched anorexia, the more I have come to realize that there is not one definitive explanation for this terrible phenomenon. My clinical experience has demonstrated, however, that it can be treated successfully and that the process of healing is quite possible. Taking into account the complexities of the disorder, the subsequent chapters define anorexia, explain it, and delineate how to treat it.

> Despite the fact that anorexia nervosa is not a condition that affects women and girls only, it *is* one that affects women and girls *primarily*, and the account of its etiology and treatment provided in this book is concerned with its specific presentation in the female population. Thus, when I speak of the anorexic patient throughout, I refer to that patient as "she." No exclusivity or contention that anorexia does not affect men and boys is meant by, or should be inferred from, this usage choice.

1

Everything You Need to Know about Anorexia Nervosa: An Overview

Definition of Anorexia Nervosa

How do you know if someone is anorexic? The first indication is physical appearance—a very skinny body, skinny enough to warrant further investigation. As a clinician, I can tell you that when you think someone might be anorexic, you need to follow through on your clinical hunch. Skinniness isn't always an indication of anorexia, but eating disorders are common enough to necessitate additional questioning. The hallmark of anorexia lies in a renouncement of eating that results in abnormally low body weight, prompted by a fear of getting fat and a markedly unrealistic perception of the body. It has been my clinical experience that it is very common for women to have unrealistic critical perceptions of their bodies and dissatisfaction with one thing or another—and, therefore, assessing for an eating disorder is largely within the realm of clinical evaluation. What follows is a composite of the numerous factors that contribute to a definitive diagnosis of anorexia nervosa.

To arrive at a diagnosis of anorexia nervosa, it is necessary to adhere to the criteria of the *Diagnostic and Statistical Manual of Mental Disorders*

(American Psychiatric Association, 2000) (*DSM–IV–TR*) for an Axis I diagnosis as part of a five-axis diagnosis. The *DSM–IV–TR* provides the following diagnostic criteria for anorexia nervosa (307.1):

A. Refusal to maintain body weight at or above a minimally normal weight for age and height (e.g., weight loss leading to maintenance of body weight less than 85% of that expected; or failure to make expected weight gain during period of growth, leading to body weight less than 85% of that expected).
B. Intense fear of gaining weight or becoming fat, even though underweight.
C. Disturbance in the way in which one's body weight or shape is experienced, undue influence of body weight or shape on self-evaluation, or denial of the seriousness of the current low body weight.
D. In postmenarcheal females, amenorrhea, i.e., the absence of at least three consecutive menstrual cycles. (A woman is considered to have amenorrhea if her periods occur only following hormone, e.g., estrogen, administration.) (American Psychiatric Association, 2000, p. 589)

In addition to the *DSM–IV–TR* criteria for the diagnosis of anorexia nervosa, it is necessary to consider additional clinical information as part of an overall understanding of the disorder as manifest in the presenting patient.

The word "anorexia" is derived from the Greek *an* (privation, lack of) and *orexia* (appetite) and is a term used to refer to a decrease in appetite or an aversion to food (Bell, 1985). Anorexia is an eating disorder identified by willful weight loss caused by extreme starvation, fear of becoming fat, and a distorted body size and image. It is a "treatment-resistant disorder," distinguished by denial (Hamburg, Herzog, & Brotman, 1996).

It has been suggested that the actual name "Anorexia Nervosa" means "self-starvation." Its Latin derivation instead implies lack of appetite . . . [but] in fact patients do not lack an appetite but instead are purposeful in suppressing their eating in an attempt to become thin. (Vandereycken & van Deth, 1994, p. 1)

Included in a criteria for anorexia are the following:

the intense fear of becoming fat, even when underweight; a disturbance in the individual's experience of her own body with respect
to size; a refusal to maintain weight that is over the minimum for
height and age; the absence of menstruation, a hyperactivity that is
paradoxical to the emaciated condition, and odd manners of relat-
ing to food. (Vandereycken & van Deth, 1994, pp.1–2)

In 1972, J. P. Feighner and associates developed yet another criteria for
anorexia nervosa (as cited in Bell, 1985). The Feighner symptoms are a
benchmark for the evaluation and treatment of anorexia and were derived
from empirical observation and statistical frequency. Included in the criteria are the following: a lack of appetite that is accompanied by a 25 percent loss of original weight; a distorted attitude toward food, eating, and
weight that overrides hunger; a denial of illness, with a failure to recognize
nutritional needs; unusual handling or hoarding of food; and an "apparent
enjoyment in losing weight with overt manifestation that refusing food is a
pleasurable indulgence" (Bell, 1985, p. 2). The weight loss and food refusal
must not be attributed to another medical illness or to any other psychiatric disorder. Finally, "at least two of the following manifestations" need be
to included: "(*a*) amenorrhea, (*b*) lanugo (soft, fine hair), (*c*) bradycardia
(persistent resting pulse of 60 or less), (*d*) periods of overactivity, (*e*) episodes of bulimia (binge eating), and (*f*) vomiting (may be self-induced)"
(Bell, 1985, p. 3).

According to Garner (2004), body image disturbance is one of the most
common clinical features attributed to anorexia nervosa. Body dissatisfaction and strong concern about physical appearance precede the onset of
anorexia, as evidenced in empirical studies. And it is interesting to note
that anorexia has been explained in terms of a "fundamental perceptual
deficit related to size estimation" and that body image is "multidimen-
tional" and involves perceptual as well as attitudinal characteristics (Garner, 2004 p. 295).

There are two hypotheses regarding the nature of body image disturbance in anorexia: One is that it represents "a perceptual body size distortion wherein the patient misperceives the actual size of her body"; the
second is that it is a "cognitive–evaluative disturbance composed of body
dissatisfaction or disparagement" (Garner, 2004, p. 296). It was Hilde

Bruch, 30 years earlier, who identified "distorted body size perception as the main feature of anorexia" (Garner, 2004, p. 296).

Bruch (1973) described three outstanding symptoms that identify the anorexic. The first is a disturbance of "delusional proportions" regarding body image and body concept. "True anorexia" is marked by the stubbornness with which thinness is defended as normal and correct and is a security against the dreaded fat. "The true anorexic is identified with his skeleton-like appearance and denies its abnormality" (Bruch, 1973, p. 252). The second outstanding feature of the anorexic is a "disturbance in the accuracy of the perception or cognitive interpretation of the stimuli arising in the body," leading the anorexic to ignore the signs of hunger and nutritional need (Bruch, 1973, p. 252). There is an absence of awareness of hunger and a marked defensiveness about appetite. In addition to denial and "nonrecognition of hunger pains," a normal awareness of hunger and appetite is absent. The third feature is a "paralyzing sense of ineffectiveness" that overwhelms thinking and behavior, which manifests in patients as feelings of helplessness about themselves—they behave in a stubborn manner, negative and defiant, and respond to the demands of others rather than behaving some way because they really want to. In the treatment of anorexia, it is only when patients have developed trust in the therapist that it is possible for them to verbalize their awareness of bodily sensations such as hunger.

Anorexics are known to fear eating and to not be able to stop eating. The "curtailment of caloric intake" is a clinical symptom of anorexia, as are odd, disorganized eating practices (Bruch, 1973). Anorexics exhibit a nutritional disorganization of eating—that is, both a denial of appetite and an uncontrollable desire to gorge themselves without the awareness of hunger. The gorging is usually followed by induced vomiting and a marked fear of having lost control. When nutritional deprivation is in an advanced state, the body is treated as if it were experiencing a famine.

Anorexics are hyperactive despite their poor nutrition, and they deny a sense of fatigue when exercising to compensate for the minimal amount food they have ingested. They use self-induced vomiting, laxatives, enemas, and diuretics in attempts to get rid of the unwanted food that may have been eaten, and disturbances in the cognitive awareness of body sensations may be responsible for such behaviors (Bruch, 1973).

History of Anorexia Nervosa

The phenomenon of anorexia nervosa in women has been around for a very long time. The history of anorexia began with women using self-imposed starvation as a means of asserting their piety. In fact, the first recorded death from anorexia dates back to 383 A.D., when a Roman aristocrat starved herself to death as a renouncement of the material world. So began the recorded history of women's use of disordered eating as a means of achieving a cultural ideal (Bemporad, 1997).

Many of the first anorexics were saints. During medieval times, female saints and mystics were "miraculously" able to survive without food and appetite (Gamwell & Tomes, 1995). The most famous anorexic saint was Catherine of Siena (1347–1380), who was known to have only eaten herbs and twigs. Columba of Rieti, a 15th-century saint, died of self-starvation by refusing to eat and actually covering her face at the sight of food. In the 17th century, St. Veronica was known to have eaten no food for three days at a time and on Fridays chewed on five orange seeds in memory of the five wounds of Jesus (Brumberg 2000). Religious anorexics of the period relied on prayer and the Christian Eucharist for sustenance.

By the 17th and 18th centuries, physicians became aware of anorexia-like phenomena among religious middle-aged women. These were known as "prodigiosa," or great starvation, and "anorexia mirabilis"—a miraculously inspired loss of appetite.

The earliest medical case of anorexia as described by a physician was cited by Richard Morton in 1686 (Bell, 1985). In his *Phthisiologia: or a Treatise of Consumptions,* Morton narrated his treatment of an anorexic 20-year-old girl, whom he described as looking "like a Skeleton only clad with Skin" (Bell, 1985, pp. 3–4). It was noted that there were no medical symptoms such as fever but a diminishment of appetite, "uneasy digestion, and fainting." The patient refused all medication offered by Morton and expired within three months. Morton was perplexed by the fact that the girl preferred to have starved herself rather than receive medical treatment, indicating that there was an emotional and psychic basis to the nervous disorder.

According to Brumberg (2000), anorexia nervosa was named and identified in the 1870s, and the "birth" of the disease in the Victorian period was reflective of changes in society at that time that had consequences for women. In Brumberg's view, anorexia is a "historically specific disease" that was the result of an economic and social environment. During the Victorian era, anorexia was a side effect of the fostering of bourgeois values that included gender and class distinctions.

Such behavior carried over to 19th-century America, where self-induced starvation was met with a public reaction of awe and fascination, and the women were referred to as "fasting girls" (Brumberg, 2000). Neurologists of the time proclaimed their disapproval of such behavior and viewed it as a manifestation of religious fanaticism or hysteria. Gamwell and Tomes (1995) contended that American society's enchantment with starvation seemed to mirror a larger societal association of femininity with madness, spirituality, self-sacrifice, and death. In the later part of the 19th century, medical professionals became aware of a phenomenon among upper-middle-class young women who fasted as a means of expressing control and power over their own lives. Women of those times had little control over their lives, so starvation and fasting became a way of exerting autonomy and, thus, rebelling against parental dictates and patriarchal control.

Before that period, anorexia was viewed as a religious phenomenon, but with industrialization, a shift took place in which it came to be viewed from a medical and pathological perspective. According to Brumberg (2000), there is a distinction between previous forms of "fasting behaviors"—as manifest by medieval saints such as Catherine of Siena—and the current form of anorexia nervosa. The saints did die of starvation, and did so by a willful refusal to eat, but they did so for religious reasons as part of a "penitential program." Brumberg has taken issue with historians who claim that "anorexia mirabilis" and anorexia nervosa were the same thing, saying that although sufferers of both eventually experience an inability to eat, the motivating factors prompting them to get to the point of becoming unable to eat are quite different. The saint or ascetic who stopped eating for spiritual reasons was quite different from the woman who used starving behavior to seek female autonomy from patriarchal societal forces.

In the case of the modern-day manifestation of anorexia, upward of 90 percent of all cases of anorexia nervosa are among girls and women (Vandereycken & van Deth, 1996). Brumberg (2000) stated that 90 to 95 percent of anorexics are young, female, and from middle- or upper-class families. Moreover, among young women and adolescent girls, there is an ever-increasing number of eating disorders, with as many as 5 to 10 percent affected. On college campuses, possibly 20 percent of female students are affected. Anorexia nervosa in boys and men presents a "different clinical picture" (Brumberg, 2000).

Comorbidity of Anorexia Nervosa with Psychiatric Disorders

Comorbidity with Obsessive–Compulsive Disorder

In addition to being diagnosed with anorexia nervosa, a patient may in fact present with other clinical disorders. As part of a thorough psychiatric evaluation, it is imperative to familiarize yourself with the comorbid disorders that appear along with anorexia. In my clinical experience, obsessive–compulsive disorder (OCD) as a comorbid condition occurs with considerable frequency. OCD is an anxiety disorder characterized by recurring thoughts or impulses that the person is unable to ignore and repetitive behaviors that intrude on functioning. Anorexics consistently manifest obsessive–compulsive behaviors, with particular emphasis on orderliness and control.

The *DSM–IV–TR* criteria for OCD (300.3) are the following:

A. Either obsessions or compulsions:

Obsessions as defined by (1), (2), (3), and (4):

(1) recurrent and persistent thoughts, impulses, or images that are experienced, at some time during the disturbance, as intrusive and inappropriate and that cause marked anxiety or distress

(2) the thoughts, impulse, or images are not simply excessive worries about real-life problems

(3) the person attempts to ignore or suppress such thoughts, impulses, or images, or to neutralize them with some other thought or action

(4) the person recognizes that the obsessional thoughts, impulses, or images are a product of his or her own mind (not imposed from without as in thought insertion)

Compulsions as defined by (1) and (2):

(1) repetitive behaviors (e.g., hand washing, ordering, checking) or mental acts (e.g., praying, counting, repeating words

silently) that the person feels driven to perform in response to
an obsession, or according to rules that must be applied rigidly
(2) the behaviors or mental acts are aimed at preventing or
reducing distress or preventing some dreaded event or situation; however, these behaviors or mental acts either are not
connected in a realistic way with what they are designed to
neutralize or prevent or are clearly excessive

B. At some point during the course of the disorder, the person
has recognized that the obsessions or compulsions are excessive or
unreasonable. Note: This does not apply to children.

C. The obsessions or compulsions cause marked distress, are time
consuming (take more than 1 hour a day), or significantly interfere
with the person's normal routine, occupational (or academic) functioning, or usual social activities or relationships.

D. If another Axis I disorder is present, the content of the obsessions or compulsions is not restricted to it (e.g., preoccupation
with food in the presence of an Eating Disorder; hair pulling in
the presence of Trichotillomania; concern with appearance in the
presence of Body Dysmorphic Disorder; preoccupation with drugs
in the presence of Substance Use Disorder; preoccupation with
having serious illness in the presence of Hypochondrias; preoccupation with sexual urges or fantasies in the presence of Paraphillia; or
guilty ruminations in the presence of Major Depressive Disorder).

E. The disturbance is not due to the direct physiological effects of
a substance (e.g., a drug of abuse, a medication) or a general medical condition.

Specify if:

> **With Poor Insight:** if, for most of the time during the current
> episode, the person does not recognize that the obsessions and
> compulsions are excessive or unreasonable (American Psychiat-
> ric Association, 2000, pp. 462–463)

It has been my clinical experience that anorexic patients present with
symptoms of OCD and demonstrate numerous manifestations of obsessions, which may include the following: constant thinking about the body

in terms of size and thinness; self-reported obsession with what they plan to eat, what they have eaten, and what foods they will avoid; comparing themselves to others (models, famous people, acquaintances, family members); thoughts about clothing size and what pieces of clothing they would wear if only they were thinner; and wearing the same article of clothing over and over again at the exclusion of another choice.

Compulsions, as prevalent in anorexic patients, are manifest in the following examples of repetitive behaviors: weighing oneself over and over again, eating the same foods, carefully excluding specific foods, methodically counting the amount of food (for example, counting out individual peas, pieces of pasta, or beans), and engaging in food preparation and eating rituals.

I had the opportunity to discuss the comorbidity of anorexia nervosa and other psychiatric disorders with Eric Hollander, a psychiatrist well known in the field for his research and practice. Hollander affirmed that OCD and anorexia nervosa are largely comorbid. He stated that for anorexics, there exists a strong need for control and for things to be their way (personal communication, June 8, 2010).

Within the category of OCDs, a "fixity of beliefs" contributes to the treatment-resistant nature of anorexia nervosa (Hollander & Wong, 2000). The symptoms include anorexics' marked preoccupation with the appearance of their bodies and subsequent behaviors that help decrease the anxieties that are prompted by their preoccupations. Anorexia patients are known to manifest an average of 10 obsessive–compulsive concerns that are not related to their weight, image, diet, or food preparation, and they experience an increase in obsessional behavior when they are starving that continues even when they gain some weight.

Comorbidity with Obsessive–Compulsive Personality Disorder

In my clinical experience, anorexia nervosa is also comorbid with obsessive–compulsive personality disorder (OCPD). OCPD differs from OCD insofar as it is an Axis II classification distinguished by "maladaptive personality features" that include a pattern of preoccupation with perfectionism and orderliness (American Psychiatric Association, 2000).

The following are the *DSM–IV–TR* criteria for OCPD (301.4):

A pervasive pattern of preoccupation with orderliness, perfectionism, and mental and interpersonal control, at the expense of flex-
ibility, openness, and efficiency, beginning by early adulthood and
present in a variety of contexts, as indicated by four (or more) of
the following:

(1) is preoccupied with details, rules, lists, order, organization, or
    schedules to the extent that the major point of the activity is lost
(2) shows perfectionism that interferes with task completion (e.g., is
    unable to complete a project because his or her own overly strict
    standards are not met)
(3) is excessively devoted to work and productivity to the exclusion
    of leisure activities and friendships (not accounted for by obvi-
    ous economic necessity)
(4) is overconscientious, scrupulous, and inflexible about matters
    of morality, ethics, or values (not accounted for by cultural or
    religious identification)
(5) is unable to discard worn-out or worthless objects even when
    they have no sentimental value
(6) is reluctant to delegate tasks or to work with others unless they
    submit to exactly his or her way of doing things
(7) adopts a miserly spending style toward both self and oth-
    ers; money is viewed as something to be hoarded for future
    catastrophes
(8) shows rigidity and stubbornness (American Psychiatric Associa-
    tion, 2000, p. 729)

In my experience with anorexic patients, many of the characteristics
of OCPD occur with frequency—most commonly, preoccupation with
perfection (that is, a perfect, skinny body); preoccupation with food in
terms of quantity and details; overconscientiousness regarding "skinny"
as a value; and manifestation of a rigid, stubborn, and willful disposition
toward eating in a disordered manner. According to Hollander (personal
communication, June 8, 2010), the comorbidity of anorexia nervosa with
OCPD occurs with considerable frequency, manifest in rigidity and a
marked need for control.

Comorbidity with Body Dysmorphic Disorder

In my clinical experience, comorbidity of body dysmorphic disorder occurs with considerable frequency in anorexic patients. I have found that in addition to anorexia, patients call attention to something additionally wrong with or imperfect about their bodies—something that is difficult for the clinician to observe but that they insist exists. Body dysmorphic disorder is marked by a preoccupation with an imagined physical defect.

The *DSM–IV–TR* provides the following criteria for body dysmorphic disorder (300.7):

A. Preoccupation with an imagined defect in appearance. If a sight physical anomaly is present, the person's concern is markedly excessive.

B. The preoccupation causes clinically significant distress or impairment in social, occupational, or other important areas or functioning.

C. The preoccupation is not better accounted for by another mental disorder (e.g., dissatisfaction with body shape and size in Anorexia Nervosa). (American Psychiatric Association, 2000, p. 510)

Patients suffering with body dysmorphic disorder are tormented by their preoccupation with and doubt about their appearance. As early as 1891, Enrico Morselli, an early psychopathologist, noted a relationship between body dysmorphic disorder and OCD (Phillips, 2000). He observed an obsessive preoccupation with deformity and a compulsiveness to behaviors such as checking one's appearance in the mirror.

In my clinical experience, patients with anorexia nervosa consistently have a distorted body image and a preoccupation with imagined or exaggerated deformity. At the very least, they are convinced that they are fat, see themselves as fat, and refuse to accept any questioning of the validity of their perceptions. There is no convincing them otherwise. In addition, there are perceived imperfections that are either exacerbated in their descriptions or do not exist at all. It is not unusual to witness perfectly normal, attractive women describe themselves as inordinately ugly, pointing out features that are the source of their distress. Subjectivity aside, they are convinced that the abnormalities exist and are angered by any disputing of these "facts."

Disturbed body image is a basic integrant in eating disorders as well as body dysmorphic disorder. Many times, anorexic patients think of themselves as fat even though they are extremely thin and obsess about their distorted body image. Eating disorders are known to manifest distortion of perception and, more frequently, body dissatisfaction. The similarity between body dysmorphic disorder and anorexia nervosa is that both have pronounced obsessive and compulsive features that are part of an obsessive–compulsive "spectrum" (Allen & Hollander, 2004).

These findings validate my clinical experience, in which obsessive–compulsive and body dysmorphic tendencies have been consistently manifest in anorexic patients. The obsessions of my eating-disordered patients have included apprehension about getting fat; preoccupation with and pronounced focus on their dissatisfaction with their weight and the shape of their body; and distress about managing their perceived flaws through diet, food management, exercise, or purging (Allen & Hollander, 2004). Even after substantial remission of their anorexia nervosa, obsessive and compulsive traits remain in patients. The obsessions manifest themselves in the form of eating rituals, exercise, or purging. Allen and Hollander (2004) have also noted that insightfulness or deluded perceptions affect treatment and are manifest in patients having either a distorted sense of their bodies or magnified beliefs about their appearance, such as the belief that others are hyperaware of their physical imperfections.

Research has found that psychotropic therapy with selective serotonin reuptake inhibitors (SSRIs) has been helpful in the treatment by reducing body image disturbances and, thus, reducing the time patients devote to and are distressed by obsessions and compulsions. In severely underweight patients, medication is not the best treatment and at times does not work because it does not help to increase weight, nor does it help in the treatment of the comorbid depression or obsessive–compulsive behaviors. In fact, the use of medication to address obsessive–compulsive symptoms and treat depression should occur only after the medical and nutritional crisis has been stabilized (Allen & Hollander, 2004).

Anorexic patients manifest an overestimation of body size that may be caused by "visual misperception," a theory purported by Garner (2004). In anorexics, size misrepresentation is based on "particular thoughts and feelings" and is a function of memory, not perception. Thus, smaller sizes are "inherently harder to estimate accurately," as in the example of how much more difficult estimating the width of a pencil is than estimating the width of a desk; in addition, body size overestimation may be an "information-processing bias that reflects a cognitive judgment rather than a perceptual event" (Garner, 2004, p. 298).

Comorbidity with Depression and Anxiety

My experience has also attested that depressive and anxiety disorders are at times comorbid with anorexia nervosa. Patients present with additional symptoms, such as those consistent with a depressive disorder or an anxiety disorder, that warrant treatment. When present, they exacerbate each other, creating a dual focus that makes treatment more difficult.

Under the heading of "mood disorders," the *DSM–IV–TR* categorizes depressive disorders, Axis I conditions, of which major depressive disorder, single episode and major depression, recurrent have the following criteria in common:

A. Five (or more) of the following symptoms have been present during the same 2-week period and represent a change from previous functioning; at least one of the symptoms is either (1) depressed mood or (2) loss of interest or pleasure.
   Note: Do not include symptoms that are clearly due to a general medical condition, or mood-incongruent delusions or hallucinations.
   (1) depressed mood most of the day, nearly every day, as indicated by either subjective report (e.g., feels sad or empty) or observation made by others (e.g., appears tearful).
   Note: In children and adolescents, can be irritable mood.
   (2) markedly diminished interest or pleasure in all, or almost all, activities most of the day, nearly every day (as indicated by either subjective account or observation made by others)

(3) significant weight loss when not dieting or weight gain (e.g., a change of more than 5% of body weight in a month), or decrease or increase in appetite nearly every day.
Note: In children consider failure to make expected weight gains.

(4) insomnia or hypersomnia nearly every day

(5) psychomotor agitation or retardation nearly every day (observed by others, not merely subjective feelings of restlessness or being slowed down)

(6) fatigue of loss of energy nearly every day

(7) feelings of worthlessness or excessive or inappropriate guilt (which may be delusional) nearly every day (not merely self-reproach or guilt about being sick)

(8) diminished ability to think or concentrate, or indecisiveness, nearly every day (either by subjective account or as observed by others)

(9) recurrent thoughts of death (not just fear of dying), recurrent suicidal ideation without a specific plan, or a suicide attempt or a specific plan for committing suicide. (American Psychiatric Association, 2000, p. 356)

If a patient fits the criteria for a depressive disorder, it is necessary for the patient to be evaluated by a psychiatrist to determine whether hospitalization or psychopharmacological outpatient treatment is warranted to treat the depression. Any suicidal ideation, plan, or attempt is in fact a crisis that warrants immediate hospitalization without compromise. When the patient is eventually released from the hospital and is no longer in crisis, it is necessary to work very closely with the treating psychiatrist if outpatient treatment for depression as a combination of medication management and psychotherapy is indicated. Compliance regarding taking medication can be an issue with anorexic patients, exacerbated by their fear of weight gain as a side effect of certain psychotropic medications. It is imperative to enlist the support of family when patients are treated on an outpatient basis, because willful noncompliance with medical treatment is a possibility to be taken seriously.

According to the *DSM–IV–TR* (American Psychiatric Association, 2000, see pp. 429–484), anxiety disorders are specific categories of mental disorder that include the following: panic disorder without and with agoraphobia, agoraphobia without history of panic disorder, specific phobia, social phobia, OCD, posttraumatic stress disorder, acute stress disorder, generalized anxiety disorder, anxiety disorder due to a general medical condition, substance-induced anxiety disorder, and anxiety disorder not otherwise specified.

In the treatment of anorexia, the symptoms of anxiety and depression are separate, coexisting conditions that reinforce the negativity of the symptoms of anorexia and, thus, contribute to the difficulty of treatment. In anxiety disorders, there is a marked hypervigilance toward information that is perceived as a threat and, without awareness, the anticipation of future negative occurrences. Depression, alternatively, is characterized by a memory selectivity that recalls negative experiences, anticipates negative experiences, and results in a decrease in positive anticipations. Both comorbid conditions can be managed with psychopharmacological intervention and the use of psychotropic medication in conjunction with psychotherapeutic treatment (Stein & Hollander, 2002).

Some Explanations of the Causes of Anorexia Nervosa

The Psychological Model as an Explanation of Anorexia Nervosa

There are a multitude of explanations of anorexia, one of which is the psychological model. Within the psychological model are psychoanalytic theory and family systems theory, in which anorexia is viewed as an adolescent pathological response to development. Starvation is a manifestation of autonomy, individuation, and sexual development (Brumberg, 2000).

From a psychoanalytic perspective, according to Sigmund Freud, an anorexic girl is afraid of becoming a woman and afraid of heterosexuality. Freud saw anorexia as melancholia with underdeveloped sexuality. Eating and appetite are both expressions of libido and sexual drive (Brumberg, 2000). In another explanation, anorexia is viewed as the inability to cope with the psychological and social consequences of adulthood in addition to sexuality and a sense of anxiety about identity. Controlling what one can or cannot eat becomes a substitute for control over the seemingly uncontrollable life tasks of adolescence (Bruch, 1973).

Additional research indicates that body image development in adolescence is critical to later self-esteem and affects the likelihood of body dissatisfaction that leads to eating disorders. Girls gain about 50 additional pounds during puberty, appearing on their hips, thighs, buttocks, and waist. Research suggests that because the weight of that normal gain is not consistent with what is considered a cultural ideal, girls experience an increase in dissatisfaction and, thus, pursue thinness. What is interesting is that although it is normal for adolescents to be dissatisfied with their bodies as they are evolving and growing, boys who are equally dissatisfied instead tend to gain weight by means of exercising to increase the size of their arms, chests, and shoulders, unlike girls, who are focused on losing weight (Levine & Smolak, 2004).

It has been found that after puberty, many girls experience dissatisfaction with their bodies even though they are of normal or less-than-normal weight, particularly because of their beliefs about the importance of body shape and weight. Furthermore, body image is the most important factor in self-esteem, and negative body perceptions are associated with low self-esteem, depression, anxiety, and obsessive–compulsive behaviors. For adolescent girls, dieting and purging behaviors are the result of dissatisfaction with their body weight and/or shape. Adolescent girls across cultures attribute blame to a "market-driven mass media" that causes the "internalization of a slender beauty ideal" (Levine & Smolak, 2004, p. 79). It is, therefore, fashion magazines, the entertainment press, and situation comedies that influence young girls with their images of thinness, a widely held ideal that contradicts what is happening to their bodies naturally. These girls are further confused by messages that encourage the consumption of unhealthy foods and unhealthy drinks, even though they are expected to be thin. Adolescent girls experience a constant struggle with the cultural standards of thinness and endless comparisons to women on television and in magazines while they are confused and dissatisfied with their own bodies on the basis of a confused sense of themselves.

It has been also suggested that the family affects an adolescent girl's sense of herself; the way parents behave and their attitudes about their own bodies influence and correlate with the body images of their adolescent daughters. Levine and Smolak (2004) indicated that teasing by family members, and specifically by brothers, has a negative effect on girls' body dissatisfaction, regardless of whether actual thinness is an issue.

Peers also have an effect on self-esteem, with girls engaging in "fat-talk" discussions in which they verbalize anxiety about gaining weight, reinforcing their sense of peer contempt. To that end, girls are known to associate with girls who have similar perceptions about their own bodies and voice similar subsequent complaints. In sum, young women are preparing themselves for a lifetime of comparisons because their bodies are meant to be "looked at, evaluated, possessed by men and, in general, treated as . . . object[s]" (Levine & Smolak, 2004, p. 81).

There is a phenomenon described by Rodin and colleagues (as cited in Striegel-Moore & Franko, 2004) called "normative discontent," in which women and girls alike regard their bodies negatively. Rodin and colleagues also found that "body image concerns" and disturbances in the perceptions, attitudes, and feelings that women have about their bodies can cause long-term psychological problems. Given that weight gain is a normal part of puberty, negative preoccupation with appearance is largely a result of internalization of thinness as a beauty ideal by the culture and, therefore, in a comparative process, girls seldom feel that they measure up to the ideal and become dissatisfied with themselves. This seems to be true despite the fact that attaining an ideal body is possible for only a few, and the greater the weight of the girl, the more likely she will experience dissatisfaction with her body even when her weight is actually within the normal range. Further, researchers have found that concern over one's body appearance actually contributes to weight increase because a cycle of dieting and purging usually follows in an attempt to control body weight (Striegel-Moore & Franko, 2004).

Evolution plays a part in explaining why women experience weight preoccupations. Beautiful women are associated with health and part of the natural selection that secures the survival of the species. Cultures that have a limited food supply prefer women who have larger bodies, yet the Western ideal of beauty is thinness. Sociocultural issues contribute to the thin ideal and present three factors: (1) the stigma of obesity, (2) the cultural idealization of thinness, and (3) the fact that physical appearance is the fundamental component of femininity. It is thinness that is held as the hallmark of current cultural beauty standards. Further, obesity is viewed as a character flaw, because it is "voluntary" and caused by a woman's failure to control her own urges. Yet there are rising cultural factors that make it more difficult for women to achieve thinness: decreases in physical activity due to increases in sedentary "leisure activities" and increases in fast food consumption and portion sizes (Striegel-Moore & Franko, 2004).

Losing weight not only alters the size of the body but—in addition, and more important—affects social status from an economic perspective and an interpersonal perspective. In response, more drastic means of altering the body, such as cosmetic surgery and similar procedures, are widely accepted because the body is perceived as "malleable" and predisposed to such alteration (Striegel-Moore & Franko, 2004). Girls learn quickly that cultural ideals are the expected standard, and "self-monitoring" and improvement behaviors are considered the norm (Striegel-Moore & Franko, 2004). The issue of body image problems for women continues throughout the lifespan and is manifest during pregnancy and the postpartum period and then again during the period of menopause. Anorexia and eating disorders are a logical consequence of the pressures placed on women to conform to cultural ideals.

The phenomenon of viewing ourselves according to the feedback we receive from others and the evaluative significance we place on the opinions of others contributes to anorexia. "Interpersonal processes" affect the process of body image development that includes a "reflected appraisal," "feedback on physical appearance," and "social comparison" (Tantleff-Dunn & Gokee, 2004, p. 109). It is the judgment of others that affects the way we perceive ourselves. Research has demonstrated that women who compare themselves with others by means of "social comparison" experience more pronounced body dissatisfaction (Tantleff-Dunn & Gokee, 2004). In particular, a predisposition to compare oneself with others is a critical factor in body image problems. Further, the more one is dissatisfied with one's own body, the less one experiences satisfaction in relationships. Anorexia and eating disorders are a logical consequence when esteem is based on the perceptions of others. The perceived opinions of strangers have an impact on body image because women conceive of how they should look according to an imagined ideal based on sociocultural directives, and these lead to increased eating disorders. In sum, body image is affected by the assessment and judgment of others and is, therefore, negatively influenced and a precipitant to image disturbances that lead to eating disorders (Tantleff-Dunn & Gokee, 2004).

Another interesting explanation for anorexia is that childhood experiences affect the ability to discern physical and emotional states. It is in childhood that one learns self-reflection and the ability to communicate feelings and experience the body through a caregiver's ability to be in tune with and respond with empathy to the child. Problems occur later in life if the child cannot develop an accurate sense of body due an inability to think in an abstract manner and is "self-referential" rather than "self-reflective." This translates into a later state of disorganization that leads to a focus on the body that manifests in eating disorders (Krueger, 2004).

In a study conducted in Australia, Mussap (2007) researched what he deemed the "motivational processes" that underlie unhealthy body changes as manifest in eating disorders among women. His findings revealed that there was an underlying sensitivity to punishment rather than to reward that motivated the desire to be thin. The manifestation of a "fear of fatness" contributed to unhealthy "body change attitudes and behaviours" (Mussap, 2007, p. 423). Mussap found that women who were fearful and risk averse were more likely to behave in an unhealthy way with respect to their bodies to avoid the negativity associated with "fatness."

Some Biomedical Explanations of Anorexia Nervosa

In researching possible biomedical causes of anorexia nervosa, I had the opportunity to ask Eric Hollander what he believed to be the cause of the disorder (personal communication, June 17, 2010). He explained that in anorexia nervosa, there is a dysfunction of the serotonin system—a deregulation of the serotonin receptors that, in his words, "are out of whack in some people with compulsive behaviors." He went on to explain that there is a possible causative link between strep infections in childhood and anorexia. He said that some of the research indicates that following a strep infection, excessive amounts of antibodies affect some areas of the brain that can later be manifest in compulsivity, as is the case with eating disorders. Such syndromes are known as pediatric autoimmune neuropsychiatric disorders associated with strep and are the subject of ongoing research.

According to Hollander, the use of SSRIs in treating OCDs, as present in anorexia, has had positive results.

Another biomedical explanation purports that anorexia is the result of deviance in biological processes generated by an organic cause referred to as "somatogenesis." In addition, endocrinological and neurological abnormalities such as hormonal imbalances, dysfunction in the satiety center of the hypothalamus, lesions in the limbic system of the brain, and irregular output of vasopressin and gonadotropin have also been found to exist in anorexic patients (Brumberg, 2000).

According to Brumberg (2000), the National Institutes of Health have reported research that found that patients with anorexia oversecreted CRH, a corticotropin-releasing hormone produced in the hypothalamus that travels first to the pituitary and then to the adrenals to make cortisol. The excess production of cortisol occurs as a response to fear and stress. Brumberg (2000) concluded that there is no "definitive answer" to the "puzzle of anorexia" but that anorexia is associated with organic abnormality, with the hypothalamus being "the most plausible site for the origin of the dysfunction" (p. 27). The hypothalamus controls homeostatic processes such as circulation, respiration, food and water intake, digestion, metabolism, and body temperature. It is sensitive to "cultural patterning," and environmental stress can result in "emotional arousal and neuroendocrine changes" and may lead to pathologic changes in the organism (Brumberg, 2002). The cause of anorexia is unclear, but three possibilities exist: (1) Starvation may damage the hypothalamus, (2) psychic stress may interfere with hypothalamus functioning, or (3) the manifestations of anorexia may be independent expressions of a "primary hypothalamic defect of unknown etiology" (Mecklenburg et.al., as cited in Brumberg, 2002, p. 27).

Somatic conditions "from blockages in the alimentary system to hormonal imbalances" cause aversion to food (Bell, 1985, p. 2). The hypothalamus controls such things as appetite, fatigue, pain, and sexual desire, and anorexics do not necessarily suffer a "loss of appetite," but they do not eat enough to be healthy (Bell, 1985).

Swedish researchers have found that female sex hormones in the womb may have something to do with the fact that anorexia is 10 times as common in women as it is in men (Procopio & Marriott, 2007). The study was conducted with 4,226 pairs of female twins, 4,451 pairs of male twins, and 4,478 pairs of opposite-sex twins born form 1935 to 1958 and found 51 cases of anorexia among the female twins, three among the male twins, and 36 among the opposite-sex pairs. The interesting finding was that in the opposite-sex pairs, 16 cases of anorexia were found among men, reflecting no difference statistically from the risk for women. The study indicated that the "shared intrauterine environment" was what led to the increased risk for male twins. Female sex hormones may influence neurodevelopment and later risk for anorexia, and males in that uterine environment would be similarly affected (Procopio & Marriott, 2007). The lead author of the study, Marco Procopio, a research fellow at the University of Sussex in Brighton, England, has warned about the dangers of anorexia and stressed that it is necessary to be aware of its early signs.

2

A Feminist Sociocultural Explanation of Anorexia Nervosa

It is arguable, from a feminist perspective, that anorexia—and the forced limitation of food intake that is its primary symptom—is the direct result of a cultural norm in which women are faced with the idealized image of an underweight, underfed, "skinny" body. Myriad books have been written about the indignity of women's struggle with weight and cultural expectations of slenderness, leading to the conclusion that popular culture and societal pressures have a causative effect on the prevalence of anorexia. This chapter is an overview of feminist writings that have contended that eating disorders are the direct result of the larger culture imposing thinness as a prerequisite to success and esteem, reinforced by the media and advertising. Anorexics, often obsessional and perfectionistic in nature, are all the more affected by the societal pressure to be thin.

In my treatment of anorexic patients, I have found it useful to introduce and integrate the feminist perspective as an explanation of the cultural issues and societal influences that have encouraged and sanctioned disordered eating behaviors. Feminist writings provide insight and clarity about the cultural norm of thinness, the prevalence of body hatred among women, and the subsequent pressure to conform. Viewing anorexia from a feminist perspective makes it possible to remove the issue of blame from the treatment and, thus, reduce patients' feelings of guilt about their purposeful starvation. As a result, it is more relevant to address the dysfunction of the behavior than it is to remain focused on—and reinforce—blame. In this reframing, the feminist perspective becomes a catalyst for taking personal action against societal forces, thus providing a shift from controlling the starvation to controlling the reaction to cultural pressure.

The mother of feminism, Betty Friedan, published her landmark book *The Feminine Mystique* in 1963, writing that women were faced with no greater destiny than to be defined by their roles as wives and mothers and noting how they became depressed when that was simply not enough. Friedan's book was required reading in my women's studies class in college, and it explained the phenomenon of women defining themselves as others' wives and mothers with no identity of their own, as if they didn't count at all. Friedan went on to challenge Freud's concept of "penis envy," which had previously been the explanation for all of women's problems and had, as a concept, undermined the strides women had made regarding their independence and identities. Friedan was particularly concerned with the influence that popular magazines exerted over women and how difficult it would be for women to deviate from the images of themselves as housewives, mothers, and objects when faced with reinforcing pressure from the media and the culture at large. She identified and defined the oppression of women as a group of individuals whose lives were determined by gender roles and limited choices. Because the oppression was widespread and not really challenged, women inherited the prescribed roles on which they based their sense of esteem and success. Thus, the emergence of the feminist movement began to challenge the notion that women's life ambitions need be limited to their roles as wives and mothers.

In *The Beauty Myth,* Naomi Wolf (1991) contended that beauty is something that women strive to embody and that men strive to possess. In post-feminist-movement times, the power structure controlled by men launched a counteroffensive to the rising power and status of women by making the ideals and prerequisites of success associated with a beauty that was attainable only through unrealistic, unhealthy eating. As a result, women were at the mercy of a beauty industry that constantly reinvented the ideals of beauty by setting standards that were nearly impossible to achieve. Wolf (1991) stated that

> for every feminist action there is an equal and opposite beauty myth reaction. In the 1980s it was evident that as women became more important, beauty too became more important. The closer women came to power, the more physical self-consciousness and sacrifice are asked of them. (p. 28)

She concluded that "you are now too rich. Therefore, you cannot be too thin" (Wolf, 1991, p. 28) and that research findings showed that successful, attractive women possessed a concealed sense of self-loathing, were obsessed with their bodies, and were extremely fearful of aging. Wolf defined the beauty myth as a political weapon aimed at subverting feminism and the advancements associated with it.

Women's identity, Wolf (1991) argued, had been "premised upon [their] 'beauty,' [causing them to] remain vulnerable to outside approval" (p. 14). As women released themselves from the "feminine mystique of domesticity," the beauty myth became a mechanism of social control. The requirement that women be thin in order to be attractive, imposed by the larger culture, was, in fact, paradoxical—albeit parallel—to women's strides in social equality. Eating disorders rose as women "breached the power structure," as a "mass neurosis" that used food and weight to "strip women of [their] sense of control" (Wolf, 1991, p. 11). Wolf (1991) stated "you don't control your body if you cannot eat" (p. 14).

There is a relationship between female liberation and female beauty, and Wolf (1991) described how women who were active feminists were thought of as unattractive and referred to as "ugly feminists." As women gained rights over reproduction through birth control and abortion, the weight of fashion models decreased to "23% below the weight of ordinary women," and eating disorders increased (Wolf, 1991, p. 11). Wolf (1991) stated that "the more legal and material hindrances women have broken through, the more strictly and heavily and cruelly images of female beauty have come to weigh on us" (p. 10). The beauty myth was a response to the cultural need to preserve men's institutions and men's institutional power.

In order to continue the oppression of women, it was necessary to refocus their preoccupation with career, competition, and success toward their perceived inadequacies as attractive, desirable women. Thus began an era in which women were preoccupied with weight—the result of a new cultural standard that celebrated unhealthy thinness. The popular culture that was evidenced in women's magazines presented fashion that reflected thinness in models and endless advice about weight loss. The number of diet-related articles rose 70 percent from 1968 to 1972 (Wolf, 1991). Without realizing it, women were faced with the prospect of reinventing their bodies and presented with images attainable only through dieting and severe weight control.

Wolf (1991) noted that research at Wayne State University found that dieting could trigger anorexia and bulimia in women who had a biochemical predisposition to those disorders. It was found that caloric restriction resulted in biochemical changes in the brain that physiologically addicted women to anorexia and bulimia. It could be inferred that societal pressures for thinness could prompt women who were otherwise normal to diet and, unwittingly, trigger a biochemically induced disorder.

Historically, women's preoccupation with dieting and thinness began around the time they were allowed to vote in U.S. elections, the 1920s. There was a rapid replacement of a curvaceous norm for women with a "new, linear" one (Wolf, 1991). Wolf (1991) noted that Twiggy appeared in the pages of *Vogue* in 1965, at the time of the advent of the birth control pill, timed perfectly to undo its "radical implications."

Among women surveyed in 1985, 90 percent believed that they weighed too much (Wolf, 1991). A "self-hatred" in women began with the emergence of the women's movement, and disordered eating was the direct result:

> The majority of middle-class women in the United States, it
> appears, suffered a version of anorexia or bulimia; but if anorexia
> was defined as a compulsive fear of and fixation upon food, perhaps
> most Western women could be called, twenty years into the back-
> lash, mental anorexics. (Wolf, 1991, p. 183)

Wolf (1991) wrote about feminism as a "humanistic movement for social justice" (p. 39). She delineated a definition of feminism that offered two differing traditions, one she referred to as "victim feminism" and another she called "power feminism." Victim feminism is marked by the viewpoint of women as powerless, judgmental of others, resentful, and "good" when compared with men, who are considered "wrong." Power feminism instead holds the view that women need encouragement to seek the power that has been denied them as a result of societal forces, which can be challenged by a responsible, collective community with an aim to make the world a just and fair place. Power feminism has among its basic convictions the ideas that men and women both matter; that women have the right to determine their own lives; that women need to be heard; that women's experiences matter; and that women deserve increased respect, education, representation, financial remuneration, and all of the things that were denied them in the past.

In 1978, Susie Orbach published the book *Fat is a Feminist Issue*, an analytically oriented discussion of how compulsive eating for women was a response to their social positions. Orbach's premise was that women were compelled to practice control over the size of their bodies and behave accordingly. She observed that Western ideals of female beauty found over-weight women offensive, challenging the popular culture's ability to make women "mere products." When women acquiesced to the mass media's view of the thin, sexual woman, they sought the "elusive power that this image promised but did not deliver" (Orbach, 1978/1986, p. 65). Women were aware that they would like to be thin and, thus, able to purchase the latest clothing and decorate their bodies in order to win approval from lovers, families, and friends. Interestingly, Orbach noted that both anorexic women and compulsive eaters shared a conscious desire not to be noticed. To that end, they were "dismissed" and were no longer considered a threat to either men or women. An anorexic was therefore viewed as one to be pitied or regarded with sympathy, but in what seemed a narcissistic attempt for "ultra-femininity," she instead desexualized herself. Orbach theorized that for some women, a wish for acceptance was accompanied by the paradox of invisibility and the feeling of "unwantedness and unworthi-ness." This "unwantedness" was the result of the implicit or explicit dis-appointment of parents at the birth of a daughter and their preference for a son. Therefore, by puberty, the girl experienced the sense of "non-entitlement" and reacted to it by refusing food, which would please her mother because she might eventually wither away and disappear. The girl was really enraged at her mother for not wanting her, and therefore she identified with a rejecting mother and responded by adopting a rejecting self-image, expressed through a refusal to accept food, the one thing the mother consistently provided. The anorexic daughter, Orbach observed, felt that she had a questionable right to survive and worried about her right to exist altogether. Orbach went on to say that for the anorexic, refusal of food was a way of showing her own rejection and, thus, demonstrating her own strength.

Orbach (1978/1986) also contended that thinness reflected fragility, caused by an anorexic's confusion about her sexuality. She explained that the upbringing of boys and girls differed in the way sexual experience was acquired and viewed. "Sex was definitely bad for girls and good for boys" (Orbach, 1978/1986, p. 176). For girls, on the one hand, sexuality was viewed as evil because they were ultimately preparing for marriage and did not want to gain a bad reputation. On the other hand, sexuality was some-thing that seemed powerful and desirable, yet was an entity that needed to be kept under control. In that confusion, the anorexic removed herself from the sexual arena in order to reduce the worry that accompanied the consequences of expressing her sexual feelings.

In a more recent book, Orbach (2001) contended that anorexic women originally sought thinness as a means of feeling more acceptable and more confident. The anorexic felt that others controlled her life, and therefore her control over food, and the ways she related to food, provided some-thing that was "uniquely her own," something that only she had control over. In her struggle with anorexia, the woman became "more in charge of her life than anyone else," and she also gained self-respect and peace (Orbach, 2001, p. 94). In her newfound strength, the anorexic became someone with no needs and no appetite. Orbach (2001) reflected on the cultural norm for women to take on the role of caretaker and attend to the needs of others, shaping their lives in the image of others at the expense of their own needs, referring to the anorexic as being on "a hunger strike in the cause of selfhood" (p. 99).

In her book *The Obsession: Reflections on the Tyranny of Slenderness,* Kim Chernin (1981) stated that "this is a book about woman's obsession; in par-ticular the suffering we experience in our obsession with weight, the size of our body, and our longing for food" (p. 1). The premise of Chernin's work brought into question the ideals of appearance for women, particularly the ideal of slenderness; women's intolerance of their bodies; and the "troubled relationship" that women have with food, appetite, and female identity. The ideal body image for women was one that more resembles an adolescent male, not a fully developed woman. Chernin (1981) provided example after example of women's dissatisfaction with their bodies, quoting one woman who said, "I've heard about that illness, anorexia nervosa, and I keep looking around for someone who has it. I want to go sit next to her. I think to myself, maybe I'll catch it" (p. 22). In her discussion of anorexia, Chernin (1981) noted that "anorexia is, after all, a condition in which mind struggles against body," that it is a "distinctively woman's condition," and that 90 percent of anorexics are women (p. 63).

Chernin (1981) pointed out that anorexia is an attempt at fighting the inevitability of the curves of a woman's body and womanhood, referring to appetite as something that needs to be controlled or destroyed. The "characteristic vision of anorexia," she observed, was one in which emaciated women felt uncomfortable with any weight gain that produced curves, reflecting a girl's fear of developing a woman's body and, thus, a woman's identity. In my clinical experience, anorexic patients express the feeling that the struggle with their body is idiosyncratic to them alone, whereas Chernin has reminded us that the struggle with an idealized body image is pervasive among women.

In 1972, Phyllis Chesler published the book *Women and Madness*, in which she explained that women were often diagnosed with pathologies that did not exist. I remember reading her book and thinking about how often I had heard references in my sessions, made by men, that women were "crazy"—the "crazy" ex-wife, the "crazy" mother-in-law, and so on. *Women and Madness* explored what appeared to be an increasing number of American women of all classes and races who viewed themselves as "neurotic" or "psychotic." Chesler wrote about the differences between women and men as therapists and how their ability to discern symptoms of being "crazy" was based on a subjective judgment rather than fact. She discussed studies of behavioral problems in boys who were referred to guidance for aggressive, destructive, and competitive behaviors, whereas girls were referred for personality problems such as feelings inferior, feeling self-destructive, or exhibiting "loser" behaviors. These observations were also consistent with the prevalence of young women starving themselves.

Chesler cited Erik Erikson's (1964) discussion of women and identity, in which he commented that much of a woman's identity had already been defined by her attractiveness and by her selectivity in her search for the man or men that she wished to be with. She also quoted Bruno Bettelheim, who said, "as much as women want to be good scientists and engineers, they want, first and foremost, to be womanly companions of men and to be mothers" (Chesler, 1972/1997, p. 112). The statements of these classical theorists supported women's aspirations to gender roles that defined their worth on the basis of their attractiveness to men.

In another feminist book, *Sweet Suffering: Women as Victim,* Natalie Shainess (1972/1984) wrote about cultural influences on women and their subsequent masochistic behaviors. Early in the book, Shainess (1972/1984) presented a questionnaire in which the initial questions include the following: "If someone bumps into you on the street do you find yourself apologizing?" and "Do you shrug off compliments instead of accepting them graciously?" (p. 13). It has been my experience that an affirmative answer to those questions has consistently been the norm with women, as has been women's dissatisfaction with their bodies, all of which Shainess pointed to as indicators of masochist tendencies.

Shainess (1972/1984) also wrote about women's cultural preoccupation with dieting and thinness and "the dictum that women must be as slender as scarecrows to look fashionable in clothes" (p. 174). She referred to anorexia as a "fat phobia" that takes the fear of being fat to a "pathological" level. Distorted body images are a prominent feature of anorexia nervosa, which, from a historical perspective, was a hysterical condition in which loss of appetite, constipation, amenorrhea, weight loss, and restless activity were the symptoms. One hundred years later, anorexia is a widespread condition, which is not surprising because of the emphasis on thinness that continues to exist. Shainess noted that eating disorders were primitive manifestations of masochistic expressions of self-hate and self-punishment, with the anorexic punishing herself by avoiding foods, using laxatives, and keeping up a level of "frenetic" activity that lack of nourishment made difficult. Eating disorders reflected the need to deal with bodily and somatic functions instead of dealing with interpersonal relations. Anorexia was deemed a masochistic retreat in which the disorder is a phobia that is self-punishing.

Geneen Roth (1996), author of *Appetites: On the Search for True Nourishment,* wrote that "there isn't an end to dealing with the longing to be thinner than you are" (p. 43). Her book questioned women's beliefs about beauty, success, and fulfillment. Roth (1996) spoke about how "you can feel the utter depravity of being in a culture that values being thin more than being alive" (p. 43) and how "the whole culture believes that being thin makes a woman worthy and being fat makes her a failure" (p. 42). She cited an *Esquire* magazine survey in which 1,000 women were asked if they would rather be run over by a truck or gain 150 pounds; 54 percent said that they would rather be run over by a truck.

Finally, in a University of Westminster in London study, researchers found that women who thought of themselves as feminists were more accepting of diverse body types and less likely to consider thinness an essential element of physical attractiveness (Nagourney, 2008). The significance of this study is that it affirmed that feminism challenged the cultural belief that thinness is the holy grail of attractiveness, a belief that has led directly to the prevalence of eating disorders among women.

3
Psychotherapeutic Models

Ideology and Choices

Psychotherapeutic intervention is a complex process that incorporates numerous theoretical bodies of knowledge to form clinical judgments. The foundation of any clinical practice is formed by the theoretical approaches that best fit the style of the practitioner and are most effective in treatment. The presentation of a psychological theory is an overwhelming endeavor, and limitations in such a presentation are inevitable. There are several theorists and theories that best reflect what I believe to be effective in the treatment of anorexia nervosa.

Carl Rogers

The hallmark of Rogerian theory is the concept of unconditional positive regard, accepting a patient without judgment, a prerequisite to any psycho-therapeutic intervention and imperative to the treatment of anorexia (Rogers, 1986/1989). Carl Rogers was emphatic in his contention that a sound client–therapist relationship was paramount to any change occurring as the result of therapeutic intervention. He believed that it is the client who knows in which direction to take the therapy, and he therefore developed a nondirective approach to treatment as a more effective means of achieving treatment success. In the early days of Rogers's career, he used an analytical approach in psychotherapeutic treatment but found that he had not successes but failures. It was from those failed treatments that he developed his nondirective approach, which was based on valuing the patient's right and ability to maintain "psychological integrity" (Demorest, 2005).

Rogers delineated three conditions that constituted a "growth-promoting" climate in a therapeutic situation. The first was genuineness and congruence. It was his contention that the more the therapist is him- or herself in the therapeutic relationship, the more likely the client will be to change and improve in treatment. Genuineness is the therapist's ability to be present in the moment with his or her feelings and attitudes. It is necessary that what is being experienced at the "gut level" is what is present in awareness and, thus, is expressed to the client (Rogers, 1986/1989).

The second condition necessary in the therapeutic situation is acceptance, "caring, or prizing—unconditional positive regard" (Rogers, 1986/1989, p. 136), the nonjudgmental acceptance of the patient regardless of what he or she presents. The therapist must willingly provide an attitude of accepting whatever is being presented, whether that is confusion, resentment, anger, love, pride, or courage. Rogers qualified this as a "nonpossessive caring." This is particularly necessary in the treatment of anorexia because the patient usually appears in an emaciated, alarmingly skinny body and is often hostile, uncooperative, and highly resistant to any attempted interventions.

The third condition, according to Rogers (1986/1989), is an "empathic understanding," the ability of the therapist to accurately sense the feelings and personal meanings that are being communicated by the patient and, in turn, communicate a sense of that understanding. It is the ability of the therapist to actively listen to the patient that Rogers considered one of the most "potent" forces for change. Rogers noted that research supports the contention that change in personality and behavior can occur when the conditions he described are present.

Rogers (1986/1989) wrote about the necessity of trust in the therapeutic situation, and the person-centered approach is based on this trust. He pointed out that this contrasts with the usual assumption that a person should be distrusted and, therefore, is in need of the social constructs and directives provided by institutions such as religion, the family, government, education, and business. This assumption is based on the premise that individuals are in need of guidance and are incapable of choosing appropriate directions for themselves. The person-centered approach is the opposite insofar as it is aimed at actualizing a person's ability to grow and realize his or her full potential. Rogers (1986/1989) wrote about a "directional flow" that helps an individual realize a "more complex and complete development" (p. 137).

Interpersonal Psychotherapy: Harry Stack Sullivan

The conceptualizing of "interpersonal psychotherapy" was the result of the theory of personality formulated by Harry Stack Sullivan in 1938. Sullivan viewed the individual as being part of a larger, interpersonal context, a divergence from the Freudian analytical thinking of the time (Evans, 1996). Sullivan's ideas differed from Freudian concepts in that he believed it was the patient's description of an experience and event that was important, not the therapist's speculations about the patient's unconscious fantasies. Freud viewed the individual from the perspective of mechanisms that were intrapsychic in nature, whereas Sullivan felt in contrast that internal psychological processes were interpersonal in nature.

Sullivan contended that it was imperative to view an individual in a psychosocial context. He was distinctive in his notion that a theory must provide scientific accuracy and must focus on the "common humanity" of which the individual is a part (Evans, 1996). His core definitions included the notion that each individual is part of a larger humanity, as reflected in his "one-genus hypothesis," in which he stresses our "simple humanity" (Evans, 1996). His notion was that all human beings share a commonality that includes biological, psychological, and social principles of life and that experience is at the core of our inner and outer realities. Thus, human experience rather than social behavior was the hallmark of Sullivan's theoretical approach.

Helen Perlman

Perlman provided the field of social work with a methodology that delineates the process of psychotherapeutic treatment. Analytical in orientation, Perlman (1957/1974) wrote that social casework is a "series of problem-solving operations carried on within a meaningful relationship" (p. 5). The end result is influencing the "client-person" to develop an effective manner of coping with a problem and arrive at a resolution. Perlman saw the role of the caseworker as that of a facilitator who helps a person understand, solve, and cope with problems, taking into account the whole of the person, which includes whatever that "whole" is, as dictated by the presenting problem. She spoke about the person striving toward life satisfaction that is thwarted by a complex of entities.

Perlman (1957/1974) discussed the engagement phase of treatment and the necessity that the caseworker comport him- or herself in a manner that portrays attentiveness, respect, compassion, and steadiness. She spoke of the importance of recognizing the individual as unique and the necessity of being open to the person's attempt to portray that uniqueness. She also spoke about an understanding of the paradoxical ability to be emotionally sensitive to the person yet provide an objective assessment of the situation and be able to appreciate the person's perspective.

Another important element of casework is the ability to enable the client to verbalize his or her problems and help provide clarity about what is being experienced in an attempt to work toward a solution (Perlman, 1957/1974). For Perlman, this is the telling aspect of the problem-solving process. She addressed the difficulty that is experienced by a person attempting to share his or her problems and suggested strategies to overcome impasses in the process. She referred to the defenses in the individual that stand in the way of self-expression in the therapeutic venue. Perlman provided suggestions that validate the client's perspective and facilitate an awareness and acceptance of whatever the client is capable of in terms of expression at a particular moment.

Florence Hollis and Mary E. Woods

Hollis and Woods (1964/1981) are known for the psychosocial theory of casework as a treatment modality with numerous specific procedures for treatment practice. Psychosocial casework focuses on the well-being of the individual and the necessity for the caseworker to provide acceptance and respect for the client's right to make his or her own decisions, a concept referred to as "self-determination."

In the treatment of anorexia nervosa, the psychosocial approach makes it possible to circumvent numerous difficulties that arise in treatment by creating an environment that lends itself to addressing the specific nature of the disorder. "Sustainment," for example, is a supportive, esteem- and confidence-building technique based on the worker's stance of projecting that the client need not be worried and can have faith in the treatment process (Hollis & Woods, 1964/1981). This is achieved when the client is presented with a therapeutic situation in which he or she is made to feel safe by the worker's ability to communicate a sense of confidence. Hollis and Woods also discussed the procedure of "acceptance," a positive communication of understanding of the client regardless of what is being presented at the moment. "Reassurance" is another of the sustaining procedures, one in which the worker provides support in the face of the client's feelings of being anxious and guilty. "Encouragement" is an additional procedure that is based on the worker's communication of belief in the abilities and successes of the client.

Hollis and Woods (1964/1981) also presented the concept of "direct influence" on the client, a notion that guidance is part of the treatment situation. They discussed the ability of the worker to distinguish the degree to which he or she can be direct and provide advice to the client and options for evaluation.

Anna Freud

I have always been fascinated by defense mechanisms and the concepts set forth by Anna Freud. These ideas are particularly helpful in the treatment of anorexia nervosa because patients are defensive and highly resistant to treatment intervention. Freud (1966) defined the term *defense* as a derivative from her father's writings to represent the ego's struggle with painful and "unendurable" ideas or affects that actually serve to protect the ego. She also spoke of an "armor-plating of character" when referring to the defenses and their use in protecting the ego from instinctual demands. Freud delineated nine methods of defense from the writings of psychoanalytical theorists: (1) regression, (2) repression, (3) reaction formation, (4) isolation, (5) undoing, (6) projection, (7) introjection, (8) turning against the self, and (9) reversal, and she added a 10th method—sublimation—which she deemed pertinent to the normal rather than to the neurotic. She made specific reference to the defense mechanisms used in obsessional neurosis, such as regression, reaction formation, isolation, and undoing.

Freud (1966) addressed the specific concerns of puberty and how the "well-marked" ego mechanisms may be magnified and more pronounced during that period. She made reference to religious fanatics and their ascetic behaviors and the reduction of food intake to a minimum as a denial of adolescent physical needs and desires. The adolescent period is filled with a fear of instincts, which are rejected by means of the defenses. One of the defense mechanisms used in puberty is self-isolation and rejection of "love objects" (Freud, 1966). In the case of the anorexic, the paradoxical relationship with food suggests a defensive stance against something that is both loved and feared.

Cognitive–Behavioral Therapy

Cognitive theory is historically derived from the work of Alfred Adler and his "individual psychology" and "holistic approach" (Werner, 1979). Adlerian theory proposed that an individual's thoughts shape his or her behavior. The implication for psychotherapeutic treatment is that by changing the person's faulty beliefs, you can consequently change his or her behavior.

To an understanding of behavior from this perspective, the concept of the unconscious is irrelevant. Cognitive theory is based on the premise that we observe phenomena and react accordingly and that faulty perceptions lead to inappropriate behaviors (Werner, 1979).

The following are features of cognitive theory (Werner, 1979):

1. Behavior is determined by thought.
2. Humans set goals aimed at informing lifestyles, and lifestyles help us realize our life goals.
3. A person's life is not controlled by the unconscious, yet it is possible to be unaware of the root of attitudes, the impressions that one makes, and the effect of one's behavior on others.
4. Aggression is not an instinctual drive but, rather, a reaction to threat or frustration and sometimes a lifestyle based on antisocial behaviors.

5. Instinctual drives do not determine or dominate one's behavior, as they can be defused or modified.
6. The sexual drive is not what underlies most behavior.
7. Thinking is at the root of emotions.
8. Motives are not unconscious but, instead, are goals or objectives necessary for our success and happiness.
9. Treatment is aimed at the thoughts, emotions, motives, and behaviors of the client.
10. Cognition is influenced by the individual's society, environment, and experience.
11. Every individual is creative by nature.
12. Change is based on modifying or expanding a person's consciousness in order for perception to approximate reality.

Beck (1967) proposed a cognitive–behavioral approach to the treatment of depression. He suggested that the patient must distinguish between thoughts and beliefs; however convincing his or her thoughts may be, there is a difference between those thoughts and external reality. Therefore, it is necessary to validate one's beliefs through an objective process in order to begin to challenge deductive conclusions and instead develop an ability to incorporate inductive reasoning.

In examining a cognitive–behavioral approach to the treatment of anorexia, Kaplan and Sadock (1989) began by describing anorexia nervosa as a "constellation of maladaptive beliefs" that resolve around the central assumption that "my weight and shape determines whether I am worthwhile or socially acceptable" and the beliefs that "I will look ugly if I gain more weight"; "if I don't starve myself, I will let go completely and become enormous"; and "the only thing in my life that I can control is my weight" (p. 1548). In their directives for treatment, Kaplan and Sadock (1989) instructed therapists to begin treatment with tasks and assignments aimed at increasing food intake and then to attempt to challenge faulty beliefs with respect to eating, how eating affects weight, the emphasis on appearance, and the "insistence on self-control." As the therapy continues, "the cognition analysis may spread out to include various beliefs not immediately relevant to [the client's] weight disorder" (Kaplan & Sadock, 1989, p. 1548).

Robert K. Merton and Self-fulfilling Prophecy

The phenomenon of "self-fulfilling prophecy" has had a powerful influence in my clinical work. Coined by Merton (1949/1968), a sociologist, the term refers to the concept that "if men define situations as real, they are real in their consequences" (p. 475). As such, the willfulness of perception as the determinant of the outcome of a situation is based on the initial expectation. This, for me, means that the mind is powerful enough to determine the outcome of a situation. If that is in fact so, cognition is the driving force that determines an outcome—what you think and how you perceive a situation has a lot to do with what it is about and whether there is a possibility for change. Therefore, psychotherapy as a treatment option would logically incorporate a way of correcting faulty cognition in order to enable change.

Elaine N. Aron

It is also important for me to include an overview of the work of Elaine N. Aron (1996) of the State University of New York at Stony Brook on what she identified as "sensory-processing sensitivity." As I researched anorexia, I came across an article by Danna Shapiro (2006) titled "Healing the Highly Sensitive Person's Relationship with Hunger, Eating and Body" in *Perspectives,* a journal published by the Renfrew Center Foundation, which is devoted to the treatment of eating disorders. Shapiro's article discussed Aron's concept of the "highly sensitive person" and how sensory sensitivity contributes to eating disorders. I was fascinated by the concepts presented and went on to research further.

Aron (1996) characterized 15 to 20 percent of the population as highly sensitive—that is, overstimulated and overwhelmed by the environment as a result of their awareness of the subtleties of their surroundings (p. xiii). In her book *The Highly Sensitive Person,* Aron included a self-test of 22 questions that provides the baseline for identifying a highly sensitive person by means of a score of 12 or more positive answers validating the criteria.

In her theory of sensory-processing sensitivity, Aron (1996) explored personality, temperament, and biochemical differences in people who possess the characteristic. Basically, people who have been characterized as introverts, shy, avoidant, intuitive, quiet, and sensitive are overstimulated by the environment. Such people possess a sensitive nervous system that provides them with an overabundance of information about their surroundings, and this can, at times, be overwhelming and difficult to process. As a result, highly sensitive people exhibit behaviors that are adaptive to their nature and consistent with sensory overload.

It has been my experience that anorexics score highly on the Aron (1996) self-test and experience the world through a heightened sensitivity that distorts and often magnifies their sense of their physical state and how that compares with external societal measures.

Family Systems Theory

In 1974, Salvador Minuchin published *Families and Family Therapy*, the bible of family systems theory. Along with his colleagues Braulio Montalvo and Jay Haley, Minuchin approached traditional psychotherapeutic intervention from a new perspective in which the individual is understood in a social systems context. Minuchin (1974) used the analogy of a magnifying lens versus a zoom lens in viewing a family and the influence of a family on its members, presenting three axioms of therapy:

1. An individual's psychic life is not entirely an internal process, influenced instead by being a member of a social system, the family.
2. Change in family structure contributes to change in behavior and inner psychic processes of the members of the system.
3. The therapist joins and becomes part of the context of the family system and forms "a new therapeutic system," and that system governs behaviors of its members.

The premise for change in family therapy is the therapist's affiliation with the family and the initiation of a restructuring process to transform dysfunctional patterns. Minuchin (1974) spoke about the formation of a therapeutic alliance with the therapist, who is positioned as a leader and joins forces with the family. The family may either dismiss or assimilate what becomes a "restructuring intervention."

4

A Multidimensional Model for the Treatment of Anorexia Nervosa

When anorexic patients present for treatment, a clinical decision has to be made regarding whether outpatient treatment is a viable option. Most patients referred for outpatient treatment have had an inpatient hospitalization, and the referral is a condition of their release. Yet there will be times when you, as the therapist, are the first mental health professional who has met with the patient, and you will be in a position to assess whether the patient is in a medical crisis or is stable enough to be seen for psychotherapy. As part of the initial consultation, you must be prepared to refer the patient for emergency hospitalization if she presents with severe weight loss, refusal to eat, and lack of ongoing medical treatment. As a condition for outpatient psychiatric treatment, it is necessary for the patient to be under the care of a physician in the event that medical issues arise. The following is a model for psychotherapeutic intervention that outlines and describes the treatment of an anorexic patient.

Engagement

From the moment that the patient enters the office, it is imperative to begin the process of engagement by providing what Rogers (1986/1989) has referred to as "unconditional positive regard," accepting and welcoming the patient as she is without judgment. The therapist must maintain a neutral acceptance of the patient's physical condition, which, in many cases, can be alarmingly skinny. In so doing, an immediate attempt is made to overcome the strong resistance to treatment that exists quite notably in anorexic patients. The patient presents with a strongly defended personal narrative, a specific story about her anorexia—the "why" and "how" of her emaciated condition—one that usually affords a limited window of opportunity for therapeutic intervention. As an integral part of the narrative, there is a marked denial of the severity of the condition. It is therefore necessary to support and protect the patient's defenses in order to begin to form a therapeutic alliance if there is to be any chance for treatment.

In the initial evaluation and intake session, the therapist must be very careful to present as nonjudgmental and unconditionally accepting but at the same time concerned about what is problematic for the patient. Part of the engagement process is to speak to the patient in a way that communicates to her that your purpose is to address what it is that is a problem for her, from her own perspective, and proceed from there. Thus, one of the first statements on meeting a patient can be this: "So, what is it that I can do for you?"

Sometimes, as a result of anorexic patients' marked denial of the severity of their condition, what is perceived as problematic by patients is not the eating disorder but the fact that they have been required to meet with a therapist. In that case, it is helpful to begin by validating that perception and attempting to make the experience a comfortable one, while at the same time asking enough questions to provide the patient with concrete evidence that there is a reason to meet with a therapist and that some good may come of the process. For example, one might intervene with the following statements: "So, you say that you spent the last two months in a hospital. How was that for you? What kind of things did they have you doing there? Did they have cable television? That must have been difficult for you. How did you end up there?" As therapists, we all develop a style that we bring to the treatment situation. My particular style is to maintain an upbeat yet serious stance that imparts a message of belief that things can improve.

Diagnosis

During the initial meeting with the patient (referred to as the "intake" or the "psychiatric evaluation"), the first order of business is to develop a multiaxis diagnosis and confirm the Axis I diagnosis of anorexia nervosa. According to the criteria for anorexia nervosa, as presented in the *DSM–IV–TR* (American Psychiatric Association, 2000), the patient should present with a history of refusing to maintain an above-minimal body weight for her age and height; an intense fear of gaining weight or becoming fat, despite being underweight; and disturbance in the way the body's weight and shape are experienced or denial of the seriousness of low body weight. As part of the diagnosis, at this time the patient is evaluated for comorbid disorders such as OCD, OCPD, and body dysmorphic disorder. In order to make a clinical diagnosis, it is necessary to carefully ask questions in a manner that is not threatening to the patient. This sometimes requires several sessions to achieve.

Evaluation

In addition to engagement, it is necessary to evaluate whether the patient is in a medical crisis and whether a potential health risk exists. Having confirmed a diagnosis of anorexia nervosa, the therapist needs to establish a baseline for weight that will help determine whether the patient is in crisis. The criteria for determining a baseline for weight should be provided by the referring medical facility or treating physician. You can ask the treating physician the weight below which the patient will require hospitalization. Inpatient facilities provide discharge reports with such information, and referring physicians can usually provide weight information. Therefore, a "danger weight"—a weight below which a patient needs hospitalization—is established as a baseline for outpatient psychotherapeutic treatment.

During the initial consultation, it is necessary to screen for and determine whether the patient is suicidal and whether there is a history of suicide attempts, ideation, or risk. It is also necessary to assess whether there is a history of depression and whether the patient has received treatment for a depressive disorder that may have included psychotropic medication at any time prior to intake.

Suicidal risk is determined by asking the patient whether she has ever thought about or actually attempted to commit suicide. Patients are usually forthcoming with such information, and being asked questions in a matter-of-fact manner is commonly met with cathartic relief. You can include the question about suicide attempts with a question about whether self-injurious behavior, such as cutting, has ever occurred. Though anorexia is a life-threatening condition, most patients do not view their disorder as a suicide attempt; rather, they rationalize that severe dieting is a means to an end and often consider thinness a noble goal. Nevertheless, if suicide attempts have occurred in the past, it is imperative to do a thorough risk assessment to determine whether the patient might be planning a future attempt. To that end, it is necessary to further assess whether she has a specific and realistic plan; if so, a visit to a hospital psychiatric emergency room is immediately warranted. The suicidal patient is not given the option of whether or not to be evaluated further; it is necessary to clearly express your concern about her potential for harming herself. You can give suicidal patients the choice of which hospital emergency room they will be referred to, and as part of the referral process, a telephone call to their emergency room of choice helps to ensure that they will be seen and have the name of someone at the chosen hospital who will be awaiting their arrival. It is necessary to contact all referring physicians in addition to contacting a family member to coordinate how the patient will be able to get to the hospital emergency room.

Assessment

It is necessary to assess whether the patient has an understanding of the seriousness of her condition and whether she will cooperate with treatment directives. Early on in the treatment, it is common for the patient to not keep consistent appointments and, thereby, make treatment impossible. With anorexic patients, it is necessary to be particularly vigilant about rescheduling and accommodating the ambivalence and resistance to treatment manifest in missed appointments. I have found that anorexic patients are willful and creative about missing appointments. Because of their tenuous emotional state, it is necessary to be very patient and understanding but firm about keeping appointments as consistently as possible. In some circumstances, referral for inpatient treatment is indicated when missed appointments reflect disorganization and mental decompensation, which can be indicative of severe pathology that needs to be addressed.

The "Language of the Anorexic"

Once the patient is engaged in treatment and is comfortable in the therapeutic relationship, it is possible to begin addressing the dysfunctional manner in which food is regarded. The patient brings with her a narrative—a personal story about the anorexia, the "why" and the "how" she became skinny. This narrative is initially strongly defended through processes such as denial, rationalization, and reaction formation. It is important to carefully support those defenses in the initial phase of engagement, with the goal of eventually reframing and challenging the logic of the patient's current state and the logic of how they became so skinny. The narrative is addressed throughout the treatment as the patient begins to accept the fact that remaining anorexic is a threat to her life and that adequate food intake is imperative to good health.

Self-report of weight can be tricky with anorexic patients because it is never surprising when their weight is misrepresented. The therapist can offer the client choices of weight measurement methods that include the following: weighing herself on a scale in the office; requesting from the treating physician the weight that was last read at his or her office; or using a piece of clothing (such as a pair of jeans) as reference, determining by sight whether they become tighter or looser as the weeks go by. (It has been my observation that anorexic patients wear the same clothing over and over again.) When the patient reports weight gain, the therapist should take the matter-of-fact stance that "this is a good thing since you are not in danger" while being careful not to celebrate weight gain and place him- or herself in the position of being the one that the patient gains weight for. It is important to affirm that self-care is the goal of maintaining a healthy weight and, to that end, to introduce the idea that "you are going to have to learn how to feed your body in a healthy way for the rest of your life, so you might as well start now."

The therapist can begin to participate in the discussion of the food paradox—the patient's love/hate relationship with food—by using what I refer to as the "language of the anorexic." Using the language of the anorexic is a treatment strategy that takes the form of an interactive narrative that incorporates an obsessional dialogue about food that is repeated in detail, systematically reframed and incorporated, in session after session over a lengthy period of time. The therapist must join the patient in the narrative, thus creating the opportunity to intervene with cognitive–behavioral methodology. Examples of the language of anorexia include the following: "So, what did you eat in the last week?" Patient answers in detail, "I ate half a diet muffin for breakfast, two pieces of sushi for lunch, and a bowl of cereal for dinner." Therapist answers, "Tell me about the muffin. What brand, where did you get it, what made you decide to cut it in half?" As a result of their paradoxical relationship with food, anorexic patients love food and love talking about food, though they fear it at the same time. Engagement in the food discussion and use of the language of the anorexic is possible only when the patient trusts the therapist and views the treatment as a nonthreatening arena for self-reflection. Only then is she able to reveal the love/hate paradox as manifest in the ability to talk about food, the perceived enemy, in any significant manner.

The language of the anorexic addresses the food issue in the following way: By joining the patient in a very personal discussion of her idiosyncratic eating behaviors, it is possible to help the patient develop a successful eating strategy. At some point earlier in the treatment, we discuss the necessity of nutritional education, and the patient must procure this information, either from a nutritionist or the treating physician. In addition, the patient is encouraged to research nutritional requirements as an addendum to the information she was already given. Together, we calculate whether a reasonable number of calories were ingested, how the patient feels in terms of energy as a result of what was ingested, and whether it translates into weight gain. The therapist can intervene through statements such as, "You ate half a muffin for breakfast. Let's figure out the calories in the muffin." At that point, we refer to a calorie book if the patient doesn't already know the exact number of calories in the muffin. We also refer to the information provided by a nutritionist or the treating physician regarding necessary caloric intake for the day. This is a tedious, repetitive, obsessional exercise and a necessary part of challenging the illogic of the anorexic reality. Again, I stress that using the language of anorexia is necessary because the patient is more likely to engage in an obsessional discussion than to just provide a report about what she ate.

Additional examples of statements in the language of anorexia are the following: "So you ate a bowl of cereal for dinner. Which cereal did you eat? How large was the bowl? Did you feel full? Let's try to figure out what full really feels like. How long have you been unable to feel full? Did your stomach make weird noises all night? Maybe that's because you were hungry. It sounds like you ate enough to feed a gerbil. What do you think you could tolerate to help your body refuel? If you were walking all day, that consumes calories, so you have to replace the calories and then some, to put on some weight. How do you think you can do that?" By carefully pointing out, for example, the fact that eating such a limited number of calories a day is hardly enough to sustain a person of the patient's height and age, it is possible to engage the patient in problem solving. In so doing, the therapist engages the patient in an exercise that will help her figure out a way to feed her body that is nutritionally sound and will lead, eventually, to the maintenance of a normal body weight.

It is particularly helpful to integrate the work of Aron (1996; Aron & Aron, 1997) and the characteristic of the highly sensitive person in the treatment. The characteristic of high sensitivity in anorexics is manifest in their perception of themselves and the environment from a highly critical stance, perceiving the nuances of body and image in marked detail. As a result of this sensitivity, the nuances resonate and are more pronounced than they are in people with a less sensitive nature, and it becomes impossible for the patient to conceive of herself as acceptable, because her perceptions are hugely magnified. From that sensitive standpoint, she imagines that everyone else is sensitive and also perceives her as less than perfect, so she needs to diet or starve herself in order to achieve that expected perfection. In treatment, the importance of identifying the highly sensitive nature is that once the patient realizes her own distinctive nature, she can begin to understand that she is more aware than others of the nuances of her appearance. It is then possible to identify and discount self-criticism and help the patient realize most of the world does not notice the imperfections and weight variations of her body and that it is because of her highly sensitive nature that she has such body image hypersensitivity.

Using the language of the anorexic, the therapist can help the patient begin to rethink her high, unachievable standards for appearance and explore more realistic alternatives to starving and unhealthy eating practices. From a cognitive–behavioral perspective, it is possible to challenge the hypersensitive behavior and help redefine a more normal standard for the patient. For example, a discussion might include a statement such as this: "No one is going to be as aware of your weight as you are (maybe a butcher might be able to figure out how much you weigh but that's about it). So long as you can think of yourself as part of a larger category of 'attractive,' you are better off concentrating your efforts on something else." We would go on to explore what that "something else" could be.

Integration of Comorbid Disorders

As part of the ongoing treatment and diagnosis, the patient is evaluated for comorbid disorders such as OCD, OCPD, and body dysmorphic disorder. In adherence with the criteria of the *DSM–IV–TR* (American Psychiatric Association, 2000) , these comorbid conditions, if diagnosed, are integrated in the treatment of anorexia nervosa. As part of the treatment, I have found it to be helpful to provide the patient with clinical explanations of the symptoms of these disorders and how these symptoms apply to them. I might delineate the definition of OCD and relate it to a specific behavior—for example, obsessive thinking about thinness and weird eating. I might point out and define the manifestation of ritualized eating and the repetitive behavior of the patient's viewing herself in the mirror at every opportunity. The same holds true for integrating a clinical understanding of OCPD and body dysmorphic disorder and how their symptoms are manifest in the patient.

Addressing Familial Issues

As part of the process of treating anorexia nervosa, the integration of a family systems theoretical approach can help unravel family dysfunction as a contributing factor to a patient's compromised mental health. Although the anorexic patient is seen on an individual basis, in the family systems approach the patient is viewed as part of a familial system. As part of the treatment process, collateral sessions including family members (always with the approval of the patient) can provide insight and an understanding of family dysfunction and possibly initiate change within the system.

Addressing "Skinny" from a Cultural/Feminist Perspective

Cognitive–behavioral therapy challenges faulty thinking, such as the anorexic patient's belief that thinness is a prerequisite to attractiveness and esteem. In challenging that belief, the integration of the feminist perspective provides an opportunity to question the validity of what has been reinforced in our culture and accepted as a norm. Feminist thinkers have written about issues such as body hatred, self-loathing, sexism, and the view of women as objects and how such issues perpetuate dysfunctional eating behaviors among women. I have found it particularly helpful to discuss, in a psychoeducational manner, the pressure that women are under to adhere to an unrealistic model of thinness and beauty. For example, as part of a session discussion, I might interject a statement such as this: "Did you know that women are exposed to 3,000 images of skinny women in the course of a week according to research done by Suzie Orbach? How can women help but compare themselves to the often airbrushed images of skinny women?" Or I might ask, "Are you aware of the historical positioning of thinness as a beauty ideal for women and how it has been a counteroffensive reaction during the periods when women began enjoying increased power and status in our culture?" By introducing an awareness of the larger issue of thinness for women, it is my intention to redirect focus from the patient's personal body obsession to a larger societal issue in which the patient is, instead, a victim. Thus, the patient begins to reframe the perception of not being "skinny"—she starts to question the unrealistic cultural standard rather than blame herself for her personal failure to look "thin enough." The eventual goal is for the patient to rethink the "skinny" standard and begin to accept a healthier, more realistic personal body ideal.

5

Case Studies

To protect clients' privacy and preserve doctor–patient confidentiality, in all of the case studies presented in this chapter, names and identifying information have been changed.

Francesca

Early in my psychotherapy practice, Francesca's psychiatrist referred her to me for the treatment of her anorexia nervosa. He warned me that hers was a very difficult case because Francesca had a long history of hospitalizations and would be resistant to therapy; she had, in his words, "hated" all her therapists and anyone who had attempted to work with her. He assured me that he would be there to supervise my work, that she needed to be seen by a therapist, and that it might as well be me.

Francesca was 21 years old, a second-generation Italian American born and raised in a predominantly Italian American neighborhood. She had been anorexic for about 6 years and had recently been released from a hospitalization. She had been forced to see the psychiatrist in compliance with her discharge from the hospital.

Francesca had been diagnosed with anorexia nervosa when, at age 15, she wouldn't eat and had to be hospitalized. She was very, very thin, dressed in baggy clothing, and had medium-length, wildly curly hair that she wore in an odd manner, covering a good portion of her face.

In an attempt to engage her in treatment, I offered few comments other than expressing support for her efforts at sharing her feelings and providing answers to my questions. Francesca stated emphatically that she was unhappy with her appearance and would not be told what to do regarding her eating. She said that she was ugly and that she was never going to get married. She went on to say that she hated her face and that was part of the reason she refused to be told what to eat—she couldn't improve her face, but she could at least have a skinny body.

At this point, Francesca's weight was above the point of crisis that had prompted the last hospitalization, but her eating was guarded, and she compensated with hours of walking to burn the calories she consumed.

During the initial consultation, although past the crisis point, Francesca was in extreme denial about the seriousness of her condition. She did not have a history of suicidal attempts ("God forbid, I don't want to go to hell. Don't you think I have enough problems?"), nor was she depressed. It appeared to me that although Francesca protested at having to participate in the session, she was paradoxically incessant in her verbalizing and had difficulty ending the session.

Francesca returned for additional sessions, speaking almost nonstop about her family's history of "weird behaviors," which were, in fact, obsessive–compulsive rituals. My work with Francesca began with the process of engagement, providing unconditional positive regard and a safe therapeutic environment. With patients like Francesca, it would be imperative to be unconditionally accepting of her appearance and to provide positive regard rather than judgment and negativity with respect to her emaciated body and questionable behaviors.

I approached this case from a structural family therapy/family systems perspective. In doing so, I was able to view Francesca as an individual who was part of a dysfunctional family system influenced by the cultural expectations that women should be thin and flawless and should consider marriage as the ultimate life goal.

Francesca was the third-born child and only daughter of a family of five siblings, with two older and two younger brothers. Francesca's great aunt resided with the family and shared her room. As the only girl in a second-generation Italian American family, much of the caretaking for both her elderly aunt and brothers fell on her shoulders. Francesca took her numerous responsibilities in stride because she did not have a choice in the matter.

Francesca was reluctant to speak about her eating habits, and we compromised that we would monitor her weight and not speak about the food until she was ready to do so. I was clear about my concern with Francesca's maintaining a healthy weight because her numerous hospitalizations were the result of severe weight loss and a life-threatening state of malnutrition. Despite her protestations that she needed to be thinner, we agreed on weighing her at every session to assess whether she was in a dangerous weight zone, as established by the discharge physician prior to her recent release. Francesca insisted that she was not thin; in fact, she was getting fat since her stay in the hospital, and everyone was making a big fuss about nothing.

Francesca spoke at length about her obsessive walking and was adamant that this was something she needed to do. From a cognitive–behavioral perspective, I challenged Francesca's belief that excessive walking served as a reasonable weight management tool. I began to hypothesize that anorexia for Francesca may have been her attempt at securing some autonomy in a phase of her life when separation–individuation was a goal that she may not have been able to achieve otherwise. In time, and as the treatment progressed, she began to modify her exercising ritual and set some limits. She was able to identify the compulsive nature of the behavior and admitted that she was often exhausted and welcomed some relief.

Although she was reticent about her eating at first, over time we engaged in a ritual of "food talk," using the "language of the anorexic" to provide an opportunity for Francesca to obsessively talk about what and how much she ate. The therapy sessions were structured to include both an opportunity for her to talk about whatever she wanted and a time for her to talk about her food intake. At the beginning of each session, we would spend the first five to 10 minutes updating her weight and discussing what had transpired during the week, and then we would proceed to speak about food. Francesca was actually open and cooperative about that. She was consistently aware of details regarding her food intake and, in time, became engaged in the process of discussing it. It seemed that no one else cared to discuss her bizarre intake of food or had the patience to listen to her detailed food narrative. The technique of joining in obsessing about food allowed Francesca an opportunity to talk about every detail of food: amount, weight, comparison of one food with another, caloric count, nutritional value, taste, the history of the food, memories of eating a particular food, and associations with the food. She was able to share her narrative about how important it was for her to be skinny and her need to be careful about her food intake.

Francesca would talk about her choice of food and how much she would eat. We would discuss together the caloric content and the precise amount that she had eaten and that she would consider eating. These discussions were obsessive and repetitive session after session. In speaking the language of the anorexic, I joined the obsessive discussion, which had shifted from a food narrative on her part to a discussion in which I was a participant. Francesca and I would talk about all different foods, sharing the commonality of Italian fare and the dictates of that culture with respect to eating traditions. We talked, for example, about the merits of prosciutto over Genoa salami and their respective fat contents. The discussions made me hungry, and I imagine that eventually had the same effect on Francesca. As time progressed, I introduced the possibility of increasing the food intake and suggested that the most important goal of anorexia recovery was the reemergence of the menses. Therefore, if Francesca were to eat in a manner that honored her body, her menstrual period would probably return, or so her doctor had told her. It was something for Francesca to look forward to. As weeks and months progressed, Francesca's weight increased slowly, with minor setbacks, but nevertheless she gained the much-needed weight.

In fact, Francesca expressed to me on numerous occasions that our food discussions stayed with her after the sessions and, as a result, provided her with the tools to challenge and change her eating behaviors. She painstakingly spoke about the efforts she made to prepare the food that she would eat. She did not eat the same food as the rest of her family, and this caused conflict at mealtimes. Francesca spoke about the non-Italian food she prepared for herself that angered her mother and aunt, who were the cooks of the family. She made herself boiled vegetables and counted them before placing them on her plate, while the rest of the family ate huge portions of pasta and traditional Italian dishes. Francesca explained that the family food choices were "fattening," and there was no way that she would eat their food. For a culture that reveres food as love, Francesca angered her family with her rejection and isolated eating.

Francesca continued to maintain that she was ugly and needed to be skinny to be physically acceptable in appearance. Yet, even in her "skinny" body, Francesca continued to view herself as "not skinny enough." As part of the treatment, session discussions would include references to feminist ideology that challenged the societal role of having to be skinny to be considered attractive. I introduced Francesca to writings that took issue with the pressure to conform to standards of body proportions that were unrealistic and encouraged body hatred. We addressed Francesca's insistence that she was ugly as part of a larger issue of wanting to fit into the American popular culture as a statement of separateness from her family, with which she had little success because she consider herself not attractive enough to do so.

In addition, our session discussions began to identify Francesca as someone who suffered from body dysmorphic disorder. We discussed the disorder at length and over considerable time, and Francesca was relieved to know that this disorder might have something to do with her chronic dissatisfaction with her appearance.

In addition, Francesca was open to learning about obsessive–compulsive behavior, particularly because she had always been labeled as "odd," being an Italian American who didn't eat enough and had weird eating habits. As our sessions progressed, she spoke about rituals that were performed by her aunt throughout the day. For example, she described how her aunt would fold and refold her (black) clothing over and over again, in a specific way, for a specific number of times. In addition, she would make and remake the bed, fold linens in a specific manner, and perform an array of random, prescribed behaviors before bed. Francesca had never paid too much attention to this behavior but did find it annoying. I began identifying the behaviors as obsessive–compulsive rituals, and thus it was possible to distinguish her eating rituals as an inherited genetic predisposition to OCD. This lessened Francesca's feelings of guilt, opening up a discussion of the behaviors rather than reinforcing the blame placed on her, as had always been the case in the past.

In our sessions, from a cognitive–behavioral perspective, we began to reframe Francesca's beliefs that "skinny" was attractive and a prerequisite to being accepted in a culture that maintains thin as an ideal for women. I challenged her beliefs and worked on increasing her self-esteem by identifying her numerous character strengths. Francesca was very bright, and we spoke at length about the positive use of her intelligence.

Throughout the treatment, I was vigilant about watching for and being prepared to identify symptoms of clinical depression, particularly since Francesca was very serious and never laughed at my attempts at humor. Nevertheless, symptoms of depression were not present, and eventually, with considerable time and increased comfort with the treatment, she began to joke about her eating behaviors and how they were horrifying to her family. She would sometimes remark to me that her mother and aunt could never understand how she could sit at the table and watch them eat foods that smelled and tasted delicious and yet remain stoic and eat the horrible "American" food. In treatment, she evolved to the point of finding that very amusing. This marked the beginning of her journey back to health.

As time went on, Francesca became well enough to terminate her treatment. She had gained enough weight to be classified as no longer being anorexic. And so she terminated treatment and, some years later, married (a non-Italian) and became a mother.

Francesca has kept in touch over the 20 years since she ended treatment and, to date, has clearly been free of symptoms of anorexia nervosa, maintaining a normal, comfortably far from skinny weight.

Cate

On a Saturday afternoon, I received a telephone call from a social worker asking if I was willing to see a patient the next day who was being released from a hospitalization for anorexia. This was her most recent in a long list of hospitalizations for life-threatening symptoms of anorexia, and the referral to me was a condition of her release. She had little choice but to agree to outpatient treatment because the insurance company would no longer pay for her costly stay in the hospital eating disorders unit. I had always been intrigued by a clinical challenge, so I agreed to see Cate, knowing that she had little interest in working with anyone.

Cate was one of the skinniest people I had ever met. Although she was "well enough" to be released from the treatment facility, she didn't look that well to me. I met with her for an intake and realized that she was extremely resistant to treatment, which was clearly communicated by her hostility. Her facial expressions and her curt answers to questions indicated that she was willful, guarded, and uncooperative.

Cate was 16 and had first been diagnosed with anorexia nervosa in the seventh grade, at age 13, when she was hospitalized for dangerously low weight and a refusal to eat. I was told by the social worker at the hospital that she was very bright and a really good student when she was well enough to attend school.

I knew that engaging her in treatment would be difficult. I asked questions but was accepting of her limited answers and general air of noncompliance and resistance. In my attempt at engagement, I tried to inject humor where possible, but Cate was rigidly immune. In my psychiatric evaluation, my numerous questions were asked with respect, neutrality, and unconditional positive regard. I managed to include questions about whether she had ever attempted suicide, and she quickly responded that she wanted to live and that I didn't have to worry about that. I was careful to provide a nonjudgmental, supportive stance, and Cate agreed to return for a second session.

During our second meeting, Cate was emphatic in her description of herself as "needing" to be skinny. In fact, she felt that she had been forced to gain "all this weight" in order to be released from the hospital and was determined to maintain her emaciated body and possibly lose some more weight. In her personal narrative, she explained that she had been "chubby" once and that would never happen again since "you have to be thin to be accepted." I listened and interjected a minimal amount but did ask her about her eating habits. She easily engaged in this discussion, providing me with a detailed, obsessive description of what she ate, morsel by morsel. It wasn't much food, but I realized that she had a need to share her obsessive eating behaviors. In addition, she insisted that she was "ugly" and not thin enough. I told her that I didn't agree but that we both had a right to our respective opinions. Basically, treatment would be aimed at addressing severe OCD and body dysmorphic disorder comorbid with the anorexia.

My one condition for treatment was the result of my concern for Cate's safety: I insisted that she maintain a weight above the danger level. She accepted that as a condition because she knew that the alternative was hospitalization. She agreed to be seen for therapy sessions weekly, expressing her feeling that the frequency would be more than what was necessary. I realized that this patient would be difficult yet desperately needed treatment for her life-threatening condition. Cate knew that too. Thus began a long, tedious treatment.

The psychotherapeutic process began slowly, allowing for Cate's resistance yet providing her with my consistent attempts to engage her and my belief that this highly resistant patient had hope for positive change. During my initial assessment, I learned that she had no history of depression, no suicide attempts, and no "cutting" or self-injurious behaviors. My initial goals were to engage her in the treatment and help her work through the issues that exacerbated her struggle with anorexia and the comorbidity of OCD and body dysmorphic disorder. In addition, it was clear to me that Cate exhibited strong denial of the seriousness of her condition.

Early in treatment, Cate spoke easily about the importance of thinness for her. She described to me her determination to be accepted by her peers, and that meant that she had to be "skinny" in order for the girls at school to allow her to sit with them at their table at lunchtime. She insisted that nobody would bother with girls who were not thin. We spoke at length about her issues of not fitting in and her difficulty forming friendships.

Cate felt that she did not make friends and did not meet boys because she needed to be thinner and thinner in order to gain acceptance. That never proved to be true, and we explored other possible explanations for her problem. Through establishment of the fact that she did have a sensitive nature and explanation of the phenomenon of being overwhelmed by her surroundings, it became apparent to Cate that perhaps this was a factor in the difficulty she had making friends and meeting boys. We discussed her shyness and her need for space and time alone. To that end, we discussed her comfort with few, yet good, friends and how that suited her nature. Therefore, it was possible to challenge Cate's belief that becoming thin would gain her acceptance and popularity. Instead, Cate needed to understand her sensitive nature and explore strategies to form friendships yet honor that nature rather than starve her body and strive for "skinny" in a dysfunctional attempt to be accepted.

In addition, as Cate's weight increased, she became focused on her "ugly face." According to Cate, there was a pronounced shape to her face that became most apparent when she gained weight, and her "fat face" was something that had always upset her. I found it difficult to see what she was referring to because she had a beautiful face that didn't look fat to me. She was insistent that she was ugly and would never find a boyfriend, let alone a husband. Cate was sure that her face was really ugly and that there was nothing that could be done to improve it; she had researched that not even plastic surgery could improve her face. We discussed body dysmorphic disorder and how perhaps these feelings stemmed from her perceptions rather than facts. Cate was somewhat open to considering a new possibility when it came to judging her "ugly, fat face."

The sessions were structured with time for Cate to talk about whatever she wanted to discuss, and a portion of the session time was spent talking about her eating behaviors. Cate quickly became a very willing participant in the obsessive recounting of the foods that she ate. Together, we engaged in a food dialogue, using the language of the anorexic in our discussions. She provided details of every morsel of food that she so much as considered eating as well as what she in fact did eat. Session upon session provided Cate with an opportunity to obsess about food, leading to obsessions about what she would love to eat and her reasoning behind depriving herself.

In the process of obsessing about food, Cate would determine the foods that she wanted to eat using nutritional and caloric information to make her choices. Cate was a master at using these guidelines because, during her numerous hospitalizations, she had received considerable nutritional guidance. In addition, Cate would weigh herself in my office weekly and share with me whether she had gained, lost, or remained the same. For the longest time, Cate's weight remained the same, with intermittent losses. Barely above what had been established as the danger weight, she was determined to prove that she could remain "skinny." I was in constant contact with her pediatrician, who assured me that she was "okay" despite her emaciated appearance.

One of the hallmarks of anorexia is willfulness, and throughout the treatment I remained mindful of that fact. One day, Cate appeared to be hiding her ankles by sitting in a peculiar manner. Since we had developed a good therapeutic alliance, Cate admitted to me that her ankles were swollen but that it was probably "no big deal." Because her personal safety was a nonnegotiable condition for treatment, I proceeded to call her pediatrician to inquire whether swollen ankles were "okay." Of course, he directed her to come directly to his office for examination, which she did, and he subsequently had her hospitalized because she had fallen below her "safe" weight of 90 pounds and was suffering from edema, a complication of the anorexia. On her release after a few days, we began challenging together Cate's judgment about food choices and engaging in a dialogue that included realistic food choices aimed at gaining weight. This was finally a breakthrough after months at an impasse.

Cate obsessed about food and, through her doing so, we identified and discussed her obsessive–compulsive behaviors. For Cate, this was comforting, because what she believed to be her own "weird behaviors" was actually something that had a name. Cate cautiously began talking more about what she ate. At first, she was vague, but within a short time she was comfortable enough to offer many more details about her food, and eventually the sessions became an arena for her to obsess with abandon about what she had eaten and what she would eat. Cate spoke about every possible detail regarding her food choices, giving painstakingly detailed descriptions of tastes, associations, feelings, and where specific foods were purchased. I would ask and she would answer, and eventually she even spoke freely and in detail about foods that she really loved but believed she probably could never eat. By joining and reframing with Cate, I found it possible to challenge the illogic of thinness and starvation and introduce moderation and healthy eating as an option.

Literally, for months at a time, sessions would include an obsessive discussion about food and choices, with an ongoing challenge of appropriateness. This would include concrete evaluation by Cate of how the food affected her weight, energy level, and overall health. During our sessions, not only was I fully aware of her involuntary need to obsess, I also willingly participate in a supportive, validating manner reminiscent of our discussions in the language of the anorexic. As a result, Cate could "think out loud" in a safe environment.

From a cognitive–behavioral perspective, session discussions were aimed at challenging Cate's logic about thinness and the cultural ideal of beauty. We spoke about the empowerment of women and the unhealthy bodies of media icons. We also integrated a discussion of cultural issues that influenced Cate's preoccupation with beauty. We discussed some feminist writings about thinness and how it compromised the empowerment of women and objectified them. Cate and I discussed books such as *The Beauty Myth* (Wolf, 1991) and the cultural importance of beauty and thinness as a reaction to the advancement of women.

We also spoke about issues such as the financial dependency of women and the importance of career. Cate was able to make the connection to the role of women in her family and their dependency on the whims of the men who were the major breadwinners. We discussed options for Cate and how she would want things to be in her future.

As a result of Cate's value system, it made sense to me that she was very impressed by magazine representations of women and fashion. She was convinced that she could never be skinny enough to be as beautiful as the models in her favorite magazines. From a cognitive–behavioral perspective, I challenged her logic and reframed the nonnegotiable standards that she held herself to. In so doing, I was able to help Cate negotiate new role expectations and, thus, be free to choose what she wanted to do.

Long into the treatment and as our work progressed, Cate's obsession and preoccupation with food began shifting to a new preoccupation with resuming her studies. We began to speak about her love for school and love for learning, which had taken back seat to her struggle with anorexia. It was at that time that treatment shifted focus from weight management to career direction, and Cate was obsessive in her ability to discuss career and school possibilities but eventually decided to enroll in college. I worked with Cate for two years consistently until her weight was out of the danger zone and she was well on her way to a normal life. One of the important concerns in anorexic women is the loss of the menstrual period. The reemergence of the menstrual period was a goal in treatment, a milestone we spoke about at length. Cate decided that she wanted a "break" from therapy, and it was shortly after that time that she called me to let me know that she had gotten her first period after many, many years, and that was a cause for celebration.

Cate kept in touch with me from time to time. We spoke about her anorexia, and she was clear that she was no longer anorexic and would never go back to "that awful period" of her life. Cate no longer weighed 89 pounds, nor was she afraid to feed her body. She reported that she continued to eat with trepidation but realized that she could not function without food. She realized that she did not have energy without food and could not restrict her food intake without experiencing lethargy and paralysis. This insight was the direct result of our work, and a direct connection was made to the effect of hunger on her day-to-day functioning. She had continued to gain weight and was of normal size, although she referred to herself as "fat."

Apparently, Cate had learned the lesson that as an anorexic, she did not have the energy to go to school, and attending school was something she really loved and wanted to do. In time, she shifted focus from her body and appearance to school and her career objectives.

Cate understood the need to shift from obsessing about what she eats to her pursuing an education. She shifted from limiting food for the purposes of body image and vanity to obsessing about her grades and studying to achieve her career goals. With insight about her behavior, she was able to channel her obsessional tendencies positively in her studies. Cate's obsessional nature will serve her well in academia, bolstering her ability to achieve high grades and pursue a difficult career with dedication and success. She has remained ambivalent about her worth as a "marriageable" woman but feels confident enough that school and career are far more important. For Cate, this represents a tremendous victory in her arduous struggle with her body.

Lucy

Connie, an obese 42-year-old, second-generation Italian American divorced single mother was in treatment with me for a depressive episode. She was resigned in her role as a single mother despite the fact that her daughter Lucy's father, her ex-husband, was a particularly difficult man and all aspects of visitation were a problem. He had a reputation for incessant telephone calling and was known to repeat conversations in painful detail over and over again. Connie was also troubled by similar behavior in her daughter, who repeated things and had quirky behaviors, such as not wanting to leave the house without looking in the mirror and completing a series of specific acts. Both father and daughter seemed to manifest obsessive–compulsive tendencies, and that was upsetting to Connie. When Lucy began high school, Connie, who by then was doing well and feeling much less symptomatic, began reporting to me that she was concerned about how skinny her daughter had become. Connie described how, during Sunday dinners with her extended family, Lucy would count the ziti on her plate and never eat the fabulous Italian pastry. She commented that she was sure that I understood since I was Italian American and could imagine how awful that could be. Connie's parents lived next door to her and made sure to point out Lucy's weird eating habits whenever they met. It seemed that her entire family was overweight, and like Connie, several family members were obese, so "skinny" was a particularly foreign concept and a cause for concern. Connie asked if she could bring her daughter in for me to see how skinny she was and to evaluate whether this was a matter of serious concern. She never referred to her daughter as potentially anorexic.

When Lucy came in for her assessment, I was taken aback by how really, obviously skinny she had become. Early in my work with Connie, I had met Lucy when she was about 10 years old, as she stayed in my office waiting room during her mother's sessions; she sometimes joined our sessions to talk about the occasional parenting impasse. I recalled Lucy as a pretty girl, of normal size, and definitely not skinny. Lucy was not very happy to join us in the session. From the first moment she entered my office, I was intent on engaging her by addressing how difficult it must have been for her to have been brought in for scrutiny and expressing that I felt it was best that we meet alone, if it was okay with her mother. Connie was fine with that but made sure to add, "Can you believe how skinny Lucy is?" (to which I made no comment).

Lucy and I spoke about everything but her obviously skinny appearance. We spoke about her comfort in her new school, her friends, her plans, her hair, and her music. I managed to ask her about her moods and whether she ever felt depressed. She answered that, sure, she felt depressed sometimes but wasn't going to kill herself and had never cut herself as many of her friends had done. I stated that if she ever came close to feeling that badly, I would really like to know about it because there were things that I could do to help. She was accepting of that statement. We ended the session by having her mother join us and suggesting that we meet again. Lucy reticently agreed that she would return.

In the subsequent session, Lucy and her mother sat together, and the focus was Connie's concern about her daughter's weight loss and limited eating. The discussion also addressed their joint concern about the intrusiveness of the grandparents and other members of their extended family. Both made comments that I would be able to understand how annoying "old school" Italian parents could be and how they should be minding their own business.

Lucy had been limiting her food intake for several months, and her clothing hung shapelessly over her emaciated body, noticeably so in recent weeks. Lucy had become obsessional in her eating, counting morsels of food and eating a very small amount in the course of the day. In addition, she would play loud music and dance for hours at a time in order to "burn the calories" of the day. I asked nonjudgmental questions about her health, and it seemed that Lucy had not had a menstrual period for several months. It was agreed that she would visit with the pediatrician before our next session, which would be in two days. I also suggested that she consider being evaluated at a nearby hospital eating disorder unit as a possible option. As had always been my protocol, both Connie and Lucy signed a release of confidential information form, giving me permission to consult with the pediatrician. Within 24 hours, I received a call from Connie telling me that the pediatrician had her drive Lucy directly to the hospital's eating disorder unit for evaluation. Within hours, Connie called me again to say that Lucy was admitted as an inpatient and that she had gone willingly.

Within four months, Connie asked me if I would be willing to work with Lucy as she was ready to be released from the hospital. She had gained adequate weight and could not be released unless she continued therapy on an outpatient basis. According to Connie, Lucy was difficult while in the hospital, gave staff a hard time, and hated all her therapists. It was Lucy who insisted on working with me, and she was eager to learn whether I would agree. This was early on in my private practice, and I was reluctant to commit to working with an anorexic patient because of the gravity of her condition. I agreed to meet with her and her mother to evaluate whether treatment would be feasible.

When Lucy entered my office, she looked pretty skinny, and I was quite hesitant to state whether I could work with her. Connie, enmeshed with her daughter, was very threatened by the possibility of Lucy working with another therapist. Lucy seemed to feel the same way and said that she only wanted to work with me because I knew her and understood her. There were issues regarding separation–individuation, enmeshment, and the seriousness of the anorexia that led to my decision to treat Lucy's anorexia in a family treatment modality.

As I knew from my work with Connie, Lucy was strong-willed and seldom did anything that she did not want to do. Connie expressed her fear that although Lucy had gained enough weight to be released, she was by no means well. The subsequent months of treatment would address anorexia within the framework of family dysfunction and resistance to treatment despite a verbalized willingness to be treated. During this period, Lucy's father disappeared from their lives, as he was known to do when problems arose.

During the first posthospital session with Lucy, we spoke about her "successful" weight, the weight that was considered safe. We established that what would be discussed in individual sessions would be confidential with the exception of dangerous behavior such as suicidal or self-injurious behavior like falling below the safe weight. Lucy had never been suicidal but did have a family history of depression that included her maternal grandmother and her mother. It was also determined that I would consult with both the pediatrician and the treating psychiatrist from the hospital, as he had placed Lucy on Prozac and would continue to meet with her monthly for medication management. The treatment plan would include both family and individual sessions.

I contacted Lucy's pediatrician, and she decided that Lucy would keep weekly appointments with her initially and, as she showed improvement, would be seen monthly. I also contacted the treating psychiatrist, who turned out to be someone of notoriety in the field of eating disorders, and I remember feeling intimidated by our first conversation. He proceeded to tell me that it was difficult to treat these patients and that if she wanted to see me, that was a good thing. He said that "she's all yours. She wants to see you and that's better than what she was doing here." He proceeded to inform me that the Prozac was prescribed to address the severity of her obsessive–compulsive behaviors, and he wished me luck in treating her.

During the initial period of treatment, Lucy and I met individually and intermittently in sessions with her mother. During the individual sessions, my focus was to engage her in treatment. By treating her with unconditional positive regard, it was possible for me to help her feel comfortable enough to begin to provide me with a narrative about her problematic eating behaviors and her intent to shrink her body. Through my remaining nonjudgmental about her appearance and accepting the obsessive–compulsive rituals that I observed—and talking with her about the subjects that mattered to her, such as friends, hair, and music—Lucy began to speak about her anorexia.

In her narrative, Lucy described in detail how important it was for her not to be "fat" like the rest of her family. She spoke about how embarrassed she had always been by her mother's appearance and how her size called so much attention to them, for example, when they traveled and her mother could not fit in airline seats. She spoke about how important it was for her to be thin because thinness was the norm at the high school she attended, an affluent, all-girl, "snotty" private school. In fact, she was excited to have been accepted at this school because of the reputation of the girls who attended it as being "the best looking girls in the neighborhood" (I actually knew of the reputation of the school from former patients). Lucy spoke at length about how she would never be fat like her mother and how she ate plenty and did not know why everyone was making such a fuss.

Connie always accompanied Lucy to her therapy appointments. On one occasion, she arrived with her own father in tow and asked if he could join the family session. With Lucy's permission, her grandfather joined the session. Connie's father was an elderly, overweight man with a thick Italian accent, and he was thrilled to be able to converse with me in Italian intermittently during the session. He had a good deal of understanding about the seriousness of his granddaughter's condition and spoke freely about his wife's depression over the nearly 50 years of their marriage. He attempted to begin commenting about Lucy's "antisocial" behavior on Sunday's and her weird refusal of food, but instead the discussion was refocused on his love and caring for his granddaughter and how he could provide help and support to her during this critical time. Lucy seemed to enjoy a positive relationship with her grandfather and expressed gratitude for my "telling Grandpa to mind his own business" about her eating habits.

Subsequent family therapy sessions with mother and daughter made it possible to discuss the difficult issue of Lucy's refusal to eat at the family dinner table on Sundays. The sessions provided an opportunity to propose alternate family plans such as eating Sunday dinner on their own, separate from the ritual of Sunday dinner with the entire extended family. In my individual sessions with Connie, we discussed strategies that would make it possible for her to eat alone with Lucy yet not experience the consequences of challenging a long-standing family/cultural tradition. We discussed plausible excuses for not eating with the family and rehearsed the probable arguments that she would encounter. Her father proved to be their biggest ally, and although he insisted that they continue the family tradition of Sunday dinners, he was not as rigid as he had been previously and seemed to acquiesce to their wishes. As time progressed, Connie reported feeling much more in control of her life and that she never would have thought it possible to not eat Sunday dinner with her family.

As treatment continued, Lucy became comfortable enough to engage in the language of the anorexic and discuss her eating behaviors in the individual sessions. It seemed that she had discovered a brand of cookies sold in a health food store that were six inches in diameter and only 100 calories. She ate three of those cookies for her first two meals of the day and some chicken or salad for dinner. It was decided that she needed nutritional guidelines so that she could feed herself in order to avoid hospitalization and forced feeding, as had been necessary in the past as a result of her condition. Lucy had met with a nutritionist at the hospital, so we decided to use the guidelines from the hospital to come up with an eating plan of her choosing.

Lucy and I discussed the eating guidelines that established caloric and nutritional intake for a day. In doing so, we began our discussions in the language of the anorexic. Every session began with a detailed description from Lucy of every morsel of food that she ate. She obsessed about amount, size, nutritional value, and her hesitancy to put food in her mouth. Hours upon hours of session discussion were obsessional, repetitive, and painstakingly detailed regarding food intake. I joined her in the discussion of every detail, examining what went into her daily caloric, nutritional ingestion. I believe that it was through my joining of the obsessional discussion that Lucy eventually came to feel a sense of control over what could be eaten and, therefore, was able to cooperate in the process of achieving a normal food intake. In the joining and engaging in the language of the anorexic, I was able to challenge the illogic of Lucy's obsession with thinness and help her develop her own ability to lose interest in starving herself and dancing to the point of exhaustion.

As the months progressed, it was possible for me to interject a feminist perspective in a cognitive–behavioral reframing of Lucy's strong beliefs regarding body image. She was convinced that "fat" was something that she refused to be. Yet, in her obsessional way, she had starved her body in an extreme attempt to guard against becoming like her family, thus asserting her autonomy in a dangerous manner. Our discussions entertained the idea that it was possible to not be fat yet maintain a healthy, normal body size without taking it to an extreme as she had done. We discussed women's images in the media and how unrealistic it was for women to maintain the bodies of magazine models. Lucy would comment on my attempted discussions of the women's movement as something that she had heard about in her world studies class. Nevertheless, the concepts of the larger culture and how unfair it was that women were held to impossible ideals were met with acceptance.

Lucy and I also discussed women's issues such as dependency and a woman's ability to be financially independent. Lucy was ambivalent about the messages that her mother had given her, the anger that she had toward Lucy's father for not providing for them, and her struggle as a single mother. We discussed the importance of education and reinforced Lucy's ability to keep up her grades despite her personal struggles.

Lucy revealed to me how prevalent eating disorders were in her school and how she was one of the few girls that did not vomit up her lunch. Lucy was proud of her position of not purging even when she felt that she had overeaten, however minimal the amount. Although Lucy engaged in obsessive–compulsive dancing, she did have an awareness of the dysfunction of that behavior. With time, she was able to cut down on the dancing and to make the connection that it had always made her too tired to do much of anything else.

A major milestone for Lucy was her preparation for the senior prom. My concern was that she would use the opportunity to backslide and return to her severe anorexic behavior. Under normal circumstances, preparation for a prom involves anticipating an event that focuses on appearance and competition. Lucy was obsessive about her choice of dress color but, surprisingly, not about her weight and physical appearance. That was perhaps because she had begun dating a cute boy who thought that Lucy was really beautiful. Lucy survived the anticipated prom event with no major regression. Not long afterward, she stopped therapy, though I continued working with her mother intermittently for a few more years and continued to hear about her doing well in college, her continued dating of the cute high school boyfriend, and her remaining at a normal body weight.

Elsie

Shortly after the terrorist attacks of September 11, 2001, I was referred a case from a guidance counselor in a local high school to evaluate a 10th-grade student for the possibility of anorexia. I was informed that the family was from Kosovo and the parents spoke little English. I proceeded to call the family and schedule an appointment for their daughter Elsie.

The family failed to keep several appointments but finally arrived for an initial evaluation. Elsie came accompanied by an entourage that included her father, her younger sister, her older sister, and a family friend. Her father spoke adequate English as he answered questions regarding his daughter. Initially, I met with the entire group but soon managed to exclude the two sisters and family friend for the larger portion of the session. Elsie was a 15-year-old, extremely thin girl who was highly resistant and openly hostile. Her father said that she was problematic to his wife because she did not help around the house with chores. He said that he really did not know why he needed to meet with me but was willing to cooperate if it was necessary. Elsie was unwilling to provide anything but monosyllabic answers to questions.

At one point during the session, her older sister knocked on the door and asked if she could join our discussion. I asked Elsie if it would be okay with her, and she answered that she didn't particularly care. Her 22-year-old sister joined the discussion and proceeded to talk about Elsie's obsession with exercise and how she hardly ate any food. Her sister had been married for several years and had a child but knew what was going on at her parent's home with Elsie and thought there was a serious problem. Elsie yelled at her sister to "mind her own business" and turned to me, stating that there was nothing wrong with exercising and that she didn't have a problem. I was careful to not antagonize an already agitated

Elsie and asked if we could meet for a few minutes without anyone else in the room.

We did so, and I asked Elsie about the guidance counselor's referral to me. She proceeded to tell me that her exercising was not the problem but her family was the problem and that she was willing to return again to speak as long as the others didn't come with her. I asked her if she was in any sort of danger, and she responded that it was the case that her family had plans for her that she refused to agree to but that she would discuss it when they were not around and trying to listen to our discussion through the walls. We agreed together to meet for an individual session, but I stated that we might need to talk to "the entourage" at some time in the future, but only if it was okay with Elsie. We scheduled a second appointment for the following week.

Elsie arrived late for the second session, hostile and resistant, and I was quite surprised that she actually did manage to keep the appointment. Elsie had really long blond hair and dressed in a short skirt that showed off her extremely skinny legs. She proceeded to talk about her sister, how she was married to a real jerk, and how that was what her family had planned for her. Her family had emigrated from Kosovo during the recent war and lived in a section of Brooklyn where there were many other recent immigrants. She also revealed that her family was Muslim and was experiencing a good deal of negative behavior on the part of non-Muslim neighbors after 9/11. She said that she did not tell anyone at school that she was Muslim because so many people were against Muslims since 9/11.

I asked Elsie about her exercising in a very matter-of-fact manner and gathered some history about her habits. Apparently, she held memberships in three local health clubs and attended all three regularly. She progressed from a hostile, guarded demeanor to an animated, highly emotional discussion about her family. She manifested severe mood changes over the course of the session but managed to provide information about the dysfunction of her family. At age 15, she was being prepared for marriage by her family, and she wanted no part of that plan. It seemed that her strange eating habits and exercise obsession had managed to stall those plans, and her oppositional attitude made her undesirable as a proper Muslim woman in search of a husband. She was proud of that accomplishment and had no intention of changing.

Elsie and I discussed whether she was or had been depressed or whether she had ever done anything self-injurious. She said that she had experienced sad and depressed moods but never as bad as the depressed moods of her mother. She stated that there was no way that she was going to get married young and never to a Muslim from Kosovo—that she would rather die than marry young. I explored those feelings and let her talk, but she was reticent, so I went on to explain that sometimes feelings of depression and frustration with things in our lives were affected by mood and that if she ever felt that badly, there were many options that could help her manage her life's problems. She went on to respond that I didn't know her family but said that she really did not want to die. Although I determined that she was not a suicidal risk at the moment, she needed to be watched carefully.

As an extension of our meeting, I asked Elsie if she would meet with her pediatrician. I had some concerns about her health because she mentioned that she also had strange, inconsistent sleep patterns that included not sleeping for days at a time. She did agree to meeting with her pediatrician, not happily, but she nevertheless consented with the knowledge that I would be consulting with her. She also agreed to return for another session.

Prior to Elsie's third session, I consulted with the pediatrician on the telephone and expressed my concern for Elsie's physical state. The pediatrician informed me that although Elsie's weight was not at the point of danger, it was necessary to keep an eye on her because she did qualify as anorexic on the basis of her obsessive exercising, eating behaviors, and low weight. I also expressed my concern for her sleep habits, a behavior the pediatrician was not aware of behavior. We agreed to be in touch and to both observe Elsie.

Elsie returned for a third session with her sister in tow. Her sister joined the session and proceeded to talk about her husband, whom she had argued with prior to our meeting. I managed to redirect the discussion to Elsie and her condition. It was in the course of that session that we discussed anorexia nervosa and how it appeared that Elsie had the symptoms. It also appeared that she had many additional symptoms, such as severe mood swings that occurred frequently and made it extremely difficult to live with her. I was interested in the fact that her mother had not met with me and that she had no intention of joining our sessions. Elsie's sister informed me that her mother had her own mood swings and was in no condition to leave the house for anything other than family outings. Our sessions did not qualify as "family outings." Elsie's mother was known to "scream and scream and scream" at home and then retreat to her darkened bedroom for days. It seemed that Elsie had some of the same behaviors in addition to her anorexia.

I continued to meet with Elsie individually for several months, during which time she maintained a low but out-of-danger weight. During our sessions, we spoke at length about her obsession with thinness and how it made her feel "American." It took a good while for Elsie to feel comfortable enough to engage in the language of the anorexic, but eventually the discussions evolved.

I used the language of the anorexic to gain an understanding of what was obviously a severe limitation of food intake and obsessive exercising as an additional means of weight control. Elsie had no knowledge of nutrition and calories and was quite open to discussing her food and learning new ways of contemplating what she would eat. What became evident was that she was eating far too little to support her exercising and that poor nutrition may have been contributing to the fact that her long blond hair seemed to be falling out. We brought this to the attention of the pediatrician, who began a treatment of vitamin injections on a weekly basis.

Intermittently during the course of our work together, Elsie would have periods of crisis during which time she would "run away" to the home of a family friend as the result of an argument with her parents. At one point, the Administration for Children's Services investigated and found that there was neither abuse nor neglect but certainly family dysfunction, for which they referred Elsie for therapy that was already in progress. During one of the crisis episodes, Elsie had passed out and was rushed to the hospital for evaluation. Fortunately, I received a call from the attending physician in the hospital emergency room, and I asked that Elsie be further evaluated for her weight and erratic moods. Apparently, she had "acted up" in the hospital, kicking and screaming and throwing things, and that was how hospital personnel learned from the family that she was seeing a therapist. Elsie was kept for evaluation and released several weeks later with a diagnosis of anorexia nervosa and mood disorder. She was referred back to me in conjunction with a psychiatrist for management of the mood-stabilizing medication that had been prescribed during the hospitalization.

Elsie met with me shortly after the hospitalization and seemed like a different person. She was lethargic and quiet and actually quite agreeable in the session. Yet something was not right, and I referred her back to the psychiatrist for further evaluation. Apparently, she had been overmedicated, and the dosage of her medication was lowered by the time I met with her again. Slowly, Elsie began to look and feel better. Yet, for Elsie, looking better was not a good thing. It seemed that within a very short time, she began to put on some weight with the medication, and although she began to look less emaciated, she began to panic about the fact that her weight was out of her control. Slowly, using the language of the anorexic, we explored strategies aimed at giving her some control over her weight.

The months that followed were difficult, to say the least, and Elsie was highly resistant and intermittently uncooperative regarding the inclusion of the medication. Fortunately, Elsie was responsive to addressing the anorexia and managed to remain at a reasonable weight as we tackled the numerous issues that contributed to her condition. Miraculously, she continued school, and I stopped seeing her eventually when she was stable enough to hold a part-time job working in a trendy local clothing store.

Sofia

I received a telephone call from a social worker in the process of discharging a patient from an outpatient treatment unit of a psychiatric hospital in Connecticut. She informed me that she wanted to refer a patient who was moving to New York City, in the neighborhood where I had my office, and asked whether I would be interested in treating her privately. The patient, Sofia, had been hospitalized several times for anorexia nervosa but had recently become well enough to be treated as an outpatient and needed to continue treatment when she relocated. Sofia was 23 years old and was moving in with her fiancé, whom she planned to marry within the year. The social worker continued to inform me that Sofia was a "lovely" patient and that she hoped that I would take the case. I agreed to see her for an intake, but the social worker insisted laughingly that Sofia would then "belong to me." I, in turn, said that I would make sure that she had a therapist in New York and that it would be me only if that proved possible. Sofia called me within hours and left several long, detailed messages for me to call her.

Sofia arrived late for the intake and was very anxious when she finally sat down in my office. She immediately stated that she "liked me" and that I was her new therapist. One of her first comments to me was an inquiry as to whether I felt that she looked fat. Sofia was of average height and quite thin, and she wore a short skirt for the intake, exposing very skinny legs. She proceeded to talk incessantly and instructed me to "write down" her diagnosis of "dysthymic disorder" and that we didn't need to talk about "the other stuff." She presented herself as what she called "a professional patient" and said that she had seen many therapists in the last few years and was prepared to tell me whatever I wanted to know. She went on and on about her move to Brooklyn with her fiancé and how she was planning a wedding. I offered few comments, was careful to respect her enthusiasm, and proceeded to ask her what she needed from a therapist. She hesitated and thought for a good deal of time before responding that she needed to fit into a small-sized wedding dress and that she had to stay out of the hospital because she had a wedding to plan and needed my help to do so. She added that the social worker in Connecticut would be in touch with her and that she had to be in therapy in New York, so she needed to find a therapist and I was "perfect." She also stated that it was important for her to work with an Italian American therapist and that she and her social worker had looked long and hard to find an Italian therapist for her in her new neighborhood. According to Sofia, because I was the only one that they could find, "God meant for you to work with me." So began a long and extensive treatment with Sofia.

From the beginning, it was clear to me that Sofia's bravado hid a plethora of problems and that the highest priority was the anorexia nervosa. In the initial engagement process, Sofia talked freely and in detail about her wedding and "the dress," and I managed to extract the clinical history and information about current functioning that I needed in order to work with her. Her social worker called me several times to make sure that I would be working with Sofia. Something about her insistence was a forewarning of a really difficult case, but I appreciated the fact that Sofia came for her appointments willingly, which was already one less hurdle to overcome in the treatment process. Initially, Sofia was seen weekly, but soon after I was seeing her twice a week.

Sofia was the middle daughter of an Italian American mother and what she described as an obsessive–compulsive Italian American father, residing in a middle-class suburb of Connecticut. She had an older sister and a younger brother living in Washington and a sister still living with her parents. Sofia had a long history of self-injurious behavior that included suicide attempts and "cutting" in addition to a history of adolescent depression. When asked about the suicide attempts, she answered clearly that they were "for effect," that it took those attempts to get her Italian father's attention ("you know how they are"), and that she had been careful to not take enough pills to actually do any harm. She said that if you said that you wanted to kill yourself, you had to be accepted into a hospital but eventually had to be released when the doctors realized that you weren't serious. She said that she definitely didn't want to die now or ever before her time ("you go straight to hell if you kill yourself"), and because she had this wedding to plan with her fiancé, Steve, who was "great," she was looking forward to "finally being married."

I addressed the hospitalizations and the anorexia, and Sofia informed me that she was currently under the care of an internist who was the longtime family physician of Steve's family and that I could consult with him freely. Sofia stated that her weight was 122 pounds and that she had gained a lot of weight in the hospital and while working with the social worker but was intent on fitting into a really small-sized wedding dress. She said that she was being very careful about her weight and would lose weight if she couldn't fit into the dress size. From a cognitive–behavioral perspective, we began to discuss her obsession with dress size. We quickly began to engage in the language of the anorexic as we discussed her food intake and her obsession with her size.

Work with Sofia was difficult. She managed to arrive late for appointments and make effective attempts at manipulating the discussions. She referred to herself as a "professional patient" many times and revealed that she had been transferred for a short time to a borderline personality treatment unit in the hospital but quickly returned to the eating disorders unit, where she remained until she was at an acceptable weight. Sofia loved to discuss her diagnoses and what she thought her treatment should be. She was reticent about her family but was clear about the fact that they were "the cause of her problems."

The session discussions were organized with Sofia speaking freely about whatever was on her mind, after which we would address her weight and engage in the language of the anorexic. With this structure, I was able to keep Sofia focused on the crisis with her eating and her history of anorexia. Our discussions would begin with refocusing from her weekly concerns to concrete issues about her food intake. Sofia shared details about the extremes she went to in order to eat her meals with Steve and yet manage to consume very little food. In fact, she began losing weight early in our work. The discussions would basically delineate the precise food that Sofia ate, and I would begin asking in more detail for an explanation of her rationale about what she chose to eat. For example, Sofia went through a period when she ate nothing but salad. When I asked if she had any idea of the nutritional value of salad and whether she had any idea about caloric intake, Sofia replied that she ate salad because it was healthy and she never gained weight when she ate salad. Sofia had little knowledge of what constituted healthy, normal eating. She had worked with several nutritionists in the hospital but did not pay attention to what they had told her because they suggested that she eat foods that she would never have thought of eating. It happened that Sofia still had handouts that were given to her by one of the nutritionists, and we decided to go over them together. Sofia was a quick learner, and we spent several sessions discussing nutrition and what foods choices were viable choices for her.

As we engaged in the language of the anorexic, we spent hours and hours discussing food choices and the value of eating a particular food. For example, I would ask, "So, what did you eat this week?" In response, Sofia would answer that she ate, for example, rice cakes or salad, and we would proceed to obsess together about the merits of salad or rice cakes and how it affected her weight, her body, and her psychological response to what she ate. As the discussions progressed, she would begin to make associations with the foods that she choose to eat, and thus we could examine what the food choices meant to her and why she had made those choices. Sofia began to understand that her food choices and limited caloric intake were about control, the control of her life that she lacked growing up in a dysfunctional household. While she was growing up, food preparation was inconsistent and many times was left to her because she was the oldest girl in the family and the natural caretaker. As we spoke about food, Sofia felt comfortable enough to express feelings that led to her bizarre choices of food. The language of the anorexic gave Sofia the opportunity to obsess in a controlled, accepting environment that allowed her to express what she had always held as a "secret," dysfunctional manner of thinking. In addition, Sofia began to discuss her father's obsessive–compulsive behaviors and understand having inherited her own obsessiveness, manifest in her eating rituals and concerns about her physical appearance.

In time, Sofia was able look back at her wedding day to Steve and comment that it seemed like a lifetime ago that she was "so skinny."

Conclusion

In all anorexia treatments, there are several themes and commonalities. As in the cases of Francesca, Cate, Lucy, Elsie, and Sofia, treatment is foreshadowed by risk, medical crisis, and guarded prognosis. Levenkron (2004) made the point that it is the therapist who is ultimately responsible for the recovery of the patient, regardless of whether there is medical support. He noted that statistics reflect a less than 40 percent recovery rate and a 5 to 9 percent death rate for anorexia. He stated that it is known that medications cannot cure anorexia but may lessen the anxiety and treat the symptoms of comorbid conditions such as depression, OCD, or bipolar disorder and, in doing so, help the treatment to progress. In my experience, it has not often been the case that medication has been used in conjunction with psychotherapy, and when medication has been prescribed, compliance has been an issue. It has been my observation that if a patient is willful about food, she will be all the more willful about medication.

Levenkron (2004) noted that there are several disadvantages for the younger therapist treating anorexia patients, particularly regarding the therapeutic relationship. These disadvantages include "the rescue syndrome"—extending oneself beyond the session boundaries—and worries about the possibility of the patient being "turned off" by the therapy. "The closer in age the younger therapist is to the patient, the more vulnerable the therapist is to those issues and the patient will see this and exploit it to 'protect' her anorexia" (Levenkron, 2004, p. 12). Levenkron (2004) spoke about the advantage of experience, saying that regardless of the therapist's age, anorexia treatment demands "more energy, patience and perspective than treating most other disorders, all the while producing the most intense negative countertransference/feelings towards the patient" (p. 12). In addition, the younger therapist has a difficult time portraying an authoritative presence. I can recall how, in my early days of practice, I envied older colleagues, felt apologetic about my youth and wished to look older to appear more credible. The treatment of anorexia is a challenge and a leap of faith on the part of the patient who, more than most, is in a dangerous, sometimes life-threatening situation.

Recovery from anorexia, according to Crow (2007), is the total absence of symptoms of the illness for a prolonged period. As anorexic patients begin the long road to recovery, I have found that, as a result of having spent so much time intent on starving themselves, limiting their food intake, and denying any opportunity to eat with pleasure, they have a marked lack of knowledge of how to feed their bodies in a healthy, normal manner. As patients begin to recover from anorexia, they begin to struggle with allowing themselves to reintroduce food into their lives, and that reintroduction opens a floodgate of anxiety regarding food. The anorexic's worst fear of losing control becomes a reality as she begins gaining weight and, paradoxically, experiencing the weight gain as success. At this point in the process, it is necessary to help the patient feel reassured that weight gain is positive, a success, and something that she can control.

The Integration of Healthy Eating and Self-Care

To further address the paradox, circumventing the seduction of dieting is an essential part of the process. It is therefore necessary to integrate a model for eating that addresses the dysfunction of the "diet" mentality as well as offering alternatives. I have found it helpful to discuss misconceptions about dieting and the subsequent psychological problems caused. What follows is an overview of what is reframed regarding "diet" behavior for anorexics and eating-disordered patients, who are consistently challenged in their ability to make healthy eating decisions for themselves.

Dieting is intrinsically destined for failure, and even though people lose weight dieting, they inevitably gain that weight back and then some more. The concept of dieting is psychologically bound to fail, yet there are things that can be done instead of dieting to succeed at managing weight. I have devised the following guidelines for weight management and self-care:

Eat Only What You Love

Not long ago, a friend lamented to me that she went on a "tofu diet" but failed to lose any weight. In fact, she absolutely hated eating tofu and ended up eating cookies to get through the day. I asked her, "If you hated tofu, why did you go on a tofu diet?" She responded that everyone in her office decided to go on a tofu diet and she too went along with it, and we laughed together as she admitted that it did not make much sense.

Diets can work for a while, but eventually one rebels and eats what one wants and, inevitably, gains back more weight than was initially lost. It is necessary to be the master of your own eating destiny. Figure out what it is you love to eat, assuming it is nutritionally valid, and incorporate it into an eating regimen. There are some serious psychological and physiological consequences to the concept of dieting. A diet is an imposed system of rules governing eating with forced limits. Following a diet may seem like a magic formula, but eating what someone else has determined you can eat rarely works. It is human nature to want to do things in one's own way, especially in the case of food. When it comes to eating—particularly for anorexics, for whom control is an issue—it is even more necessary to make one's own choices. If you are told what to eat and it's not something that you like, it is just a matter of time until you will give up and return to familiar food choices. What works for one person does not necessarily work for another person; therefore, it is necessary to come up with a customized eating strategy that takes into account what it takes for you to feel satisfied. An eating plan is only as good as the person whom the plan is for is motivated to follow it. So, figure out the things that you really love to eat in the course of a day and . . .

Become Informed about Calories and Nutrition

I had a friend during college who had health issues and needed to lose weight. As friends do, she talked me into going to a Weight Watchers meeting with her (I had the car). I was allowed to sit with her during the meeting as long as I participated. It sounded like fun since the meeting was about food—lists and lists of foods you could eat, even foods I never thought of eating. So I went home and ate some cool new foods. I went back with her the next week and even weighed myself. I had gained three pounds, and the leader asked me to speak to her after the meeting. Well, that was it for Weight Watchers and me in the 70s, but I did learn one thing—it helps to know calories. With the knowledge of calories, you will have the ability to choose lower calorie foods to substitute for higher calorie foods. Low-calorie food substitutions will help you manage hunger and limit excessive eating, which is the key to weight loss and management.

Knowledge of calories is particularly worth acquiring for recovering anorexia patients. As a result of the obsessiveness of their nature, they are inclined to measure and regulate their food intake anyway. With the knowledge of calories comes the ability to make informed decisions about what foods and how much of them should be eaten. Many times anorexics have no idea of how truly minimal their caloric intake is because they dramatically overestimate the amount of food that they eat. They will insist that they ate plenty when in fact they ate "gerbil portions" of food.

The counting of calories is inarguable—objective—and helps inform the process of increasing food intake in order to reach a normal weight. It is possible to calculate how many daily calories are required to maintain a healthy weight and launch a discussion of how to achieve that optimal level of food intake. I have found it helpful to incorporate the exercise of reading food labels so that patients are empowered to eat in an informed manner rather than on the basis of faulty fears of weight gain. Procuring nutritional information helps them to make informed and appropriate eating choices in the service of realizing a healthy weight.

Learn to Eat in Moderation

Years ago, I remember buying a frozen entrée of ravioli, and, after waiting 45 minutes while it heated in the toaster oven, when it was finally ready to eat, I was shocked to see only three pitiful ravioli staring at me. I impatiently grabbed the box to find the customer service telephone number, dialed it, and complained that the box I purchased had not been properly filled with food. To my surprise, I was told that this was the correct portion. I was amazed that anybody could consider three ravioli a meal.

Satiety is an important part of eating. Sometimes, establishing reasonable portions of food requires thought and creativity to allow one to experience the feeling of having eaten enough. The fear in anorexic patients is that they will go overboard and gain an uncontrollable amount of weight when left to their own devices, particularly because they have starved themselves and are chronically hungry. And, in fact, many times anorexics do engage in binge eating after a prolonged period of starvation. By learning how to eat to the point of respecting what the body actually needs to feel full, recovering anorexics exercise the ability to control what they eat and how much, thus avoiding fear and need to binge. Anorexics have learned to ignore hunger and, consequently, have no idea when they are full. This is a complicated process that takes time and patience to learn. Anorexics all too often need to relearn how to eat enough to gain and maintain a healthy body weight. Learning to eat in moderation addresses their need for control yet helps establish a lifetime habit of self-care.

Understand Eating as a Behavior of Habit

People eat what they are used to eating. Most favorite foods are chosen out of habit. Habits are behaviors that become automatic over time and consequently take considerable motivation and time to change. To change eating habits, it is necessary to begin substituting satisfying food choices for unhealthy ones, thus establishing a new habit in place of an old, faulty one. Making food-choice decisions begins the process of empowerment, coupled with awareness of the fact that it will take time to change a habit.

Make Peace with Your Body

An exercise I give my patients is one in which they challenge their obsessional, perfectionistic behavior with respect to their critical judgment of their body and appearance. I ask them to begin making a mental note of how often they judge the appearance of others, beginning the moment they leave my office. How often do we look at others and have a critical judgment such as "How can that person wear that hat?" or "That person looks so bad" or ". . . so overweight" or ". . . so skinny"? I remind my patients that women are often guilty of the "once over" behavior that has us comparing ourselves to other women, real women or magazine images, and how that is a losing proposition because there will always be prettier women or younger women or thinner women. I ask them to temper that judgment with a more accepting stance, such as "That person looks fine" or "That person looks great." As patients do this exercise, they begin to realize that the perception that other people are judging them stems from their own judgmental behavior—behavior that needs to be challenged. In challenging it, they will begin to be more accepting of themselves and others. And further, with respect to self-acceptance, I remind women to do the best that they can to take care of themselves in terms of grooming and exercise and to wear only things that make them feel good. With time, the habit of self-criticism begins being replaced by self-acceptance.

It is necessary to make peace with one's body. We are living in a time of major preoccupation with personal appearance, evident in the popularity of reality television "makeover" programs. There is a difference between self-improvement and change motivated by self-loathing or a distorted body image. It is imperative to have an accepting attitude toward one's own body. To this end, I give my patients another exercise that consists of going home and looking at their bodies in a mirror in a loving manner. Inevitably, this exercise is met with horror, apprehension, and laughter. Never has anyone returned with the comment, "I look great" or "I love the way I look." It is really sad to validate Orbach's (2008) statement that 98 percent of women do not think of themselves as beautiful when beauty is the pinnacle of women's existence, according to our culture.

More important than how you look is that your body can function and is healthy. Women are influenced by popular culture and really do not stand a chance of measuring up to a standard that is inconsistent and subjective. No one's body is perfect, and women largely exaggerate their flaws. We're rarely happy with the way we look, but it's really okay to look less than perfect. Beauty lies in feeling good about yourself as you are now. And you really are more important than how you look. The key to making peace with one's body is to understand and accept that we're all trying to cope with life in the best way that we can, and that is no small task. With some effort, it is possible to better manage one's eating. By initiating a discussion about making peace with your body, it is possible to begin a dialogue about the upward struggle between self-acceptance and self-care.

Change is always possible.

References

Allen, A., & Hollander, E. (2004). Psychopharmacological treatments for body image disturbances. In T. F. Cash & T. Pruzinsky (Eds.), *Body image: A handbook of theory, research, and clinical practice* (pp. 450–458). New York: Guilford Press.

American Psychiatric Association. (2000). *Diagnostic and statistical manual of mental disorders* (4th ed., text rev.). Washington, DC: Author.

Aron, E. N. (1996). *The highly sensitive person: How to thrive when the world overwhelms you.* New York: Broadway Books.

Aron, E. N., & Aron, A. (1997). Sensory-processing sensitivity and its relation to introversion and emotionality. *Journal of Personality and Social Psychology, 73,* 345–368.

Beck, A. T. (1967). *Depression causes and treatment.* Philadelphia: University of Pennsylvania Press.

Bell, R. M. (1985). *Holy anorexia.* Chicago: University of Chicago Press.

Bemporad, J. R. (1997, September). The prehistory of anorexia nervosa. *Newsletter of the Psychosomatic Discussion Group of the American Psychoanalytic Association.* Retrieved from http://www.cyberpsych.org/pdg/pdghist.htm

Bruch, H. (1973). *Eating disorders: Obesity, anorexia nervosa, and the person within.* New York: Basic Books.

Brumberg, J. J. (2000). *Fasting girls: The history of anorexia nervosa.* New York: Vintage Books.

Chernin, K. (1981). *The obsession: Reflections on the tyranny of slenderness.* New York: Harper & Row.

Chesler, P. (1997). *Women and madness.* New York: Four Walls Eight Windows. (Original work published 1972)

Crow, S. (2007, Winter). Recovery from eating disorders. *Perspectives: A Professional Journal of the Renfrew Center Foundation, 12,* 1–3.

Demorest, A. (2005). *Psychology's grand theorists: How personal experience shaped professional ideas.* Mahwah, NJ: Lawrence Erlbaum Associates.

Erikson, E. (1964). Inner and outer space: Reflections on womanhood. *Daedalus*(3), 582–606.

Evans, F. B., III. (1996). *Harry Stack Sullivan: Interpersonal theory and psychotherapy.* London: Routledge.

Freud, A. (1966). *The ego and the mechanisms of defense: The writings of Anna Freud, vol. 2* (Rev. ed.). New York: International Universities Press.

Friedan, B. (1963). *The feminine mystique.* New York: Dell.

Freedman, R., & Barnouvin, K. (2005). *Skinny bitch: A no-nonsense, tough-love guide for savvy girls who want to stop eating crap and start looking fabulous!* Philadelphia: Running Press.

Gamwell, L., & Tomes, N. (1995). *Madness in America: Cultural and medical perceptions of mental illness before 1914.* Ithaca, NY: Cornell University Press.

Garner, D. M. (2004). Body image and anorexia nervosa. In T. F. Cash & T. Pruzinsky (Eds.), *Body image: A handbook of theory, research, and clinical practice* (pp. 295–303). New York: Guilford Press.

Hamburg, P., Herzog, D. B., & Brotman, A. (1996). Treatment resistance in eating disorders: Psychodynamic and pharmacologic perspectives. In M. H. Pollack, M. W.Otto, & J. F. Rosenbaum (Eds.), *Challenges in clinical practice* (pp. 263–275). New York: Guilford Press.

Hollander, E., & Wong, C. M. (2000). Spectrum, boundary, and subtyping issues: Implications for treatment-refractory obsessive–compulsive disorder. In W. K. Goodman, M. V. Rudorfer, & J. D. Maser (Eds.) *Obsessive–compulsive disorder: Contemporary treatment issues* (pp. 3–22). Mahwah, NJ: Lawrence Erlbaum Associates.

Hollis, F., & Woods, M. E. (1981). *Casework: A psychosocial therapy* (3rd ed.). New York: Random House. (Original work published 1964)

Kaplan, H. I., & Sadock, B. J. (1989). *Comprehensive textbook of psychiatry* (5th ed., Vol. 2). Baltimore: Williams & Wilkins.

Krueger, D. W. (2004). Psychodynamic approaches to changing body image. In T. F. Cash & T. Pruzinsky, *Body image: A handbook of theory, research, and clinical practice* (pp. 30–37). New York: Guilford Press.

Levenkron, S. (2004, Summer). Younger and older: The therapist's age as a factor in treating anorexia. *Perspectives: A Professional Journal of the Renfrew Center Foundation, 9,* 12–13.

Levine, M. P., & Smolak, L. (2004). Body image development in adolescence. In T. F. Cash & T. Pruzinsky (Eds.), *Body image: A handbook of theory, research, and clinical practice* (pp. 74–82). New York: Guilford Press.

Merton, R. K. (1968). *Social theory and social structure.* New York: Free Press. (Original work published 1949)

Minuchin, S. (1974). *Families and family therapy.* Cambridge, MA: Harvard University Press.

Mussap, A. J. (2007). Motivational processes associated with unhealthy body change attitudes and behaviours. *Eating Behaviours, 8,* 423–428.

Nagourney, E. (2008, March 25). Perceptions: Feminists more open-minded on weight. *New York Times.* Retrieved from http://www.nytimes.com/2008/03/25/health/research/25perc.html

Orbach, S. (1986). *Fat is a feminist issue: A self-help guide for compulsive eaters.* New York: Berkley Books. (Original work published 1978)

Orbach, S. (2001). *Hunger strike: Starving amidst plenty.* New York: Other Press.

Orbach, S. (2008, March 8). Contribution to the proceedings of Indwelling II: Living in a Female Body: The Project Continues, New York.

Perlman, H. H. (1974). *Social casework: A problem-solving process.* Chicago: University of Chicago Press. (Original work published 1957)

Phillips, K. A. (2000). Connection between obsessive–compulsive disorder and body dysmorphic disorder. In W. K. Goodman, M. V. Rudorfer, & J. D. Maser (Eds.), *Obsessive–compulsive disorder: Contemporary issues in treatment* (pp. 23–42). Mahwah, NJ: Lawrence Erlbaum Associates.

Procopio, M., & Marriott, P. (2007). Intrauterine hormonal environment and risk of developing anorexia nervosa. *Archives of General Psychiatry, 64,* 1402–1407.

Rogers, C. (1989). A client-centered/person-centered approach to therapy. In H. Kirschnbaum & V. L. Henderson (Eds.), *The Carl Rogers reader* (pp. 135–152). Boston: Houghton Mifflin. (Original work published 1986)

Roth, G. (1996). *Appetites: On the search for true nourishment.* New York: Dutton.

Shainess, N. (1984). *Sweet suffering: Woman as victim.* New York: Bobbs-Merrill. (Original work published 1972)

Shapiro, D. (2006, Summer). Healing the highly sensitive person's relationship with hunger, eating and body. *Perspectives: A Professional Journal of the Renfrew Center Foundation, 11,* 20–21.

Shaw, G. (2005). *Anorexia: The body neglected.* Retrieved from http://www.webmd.com/mental-health/anorexia-nervosa/features/anorexia-body-neglected

Stein, D. J., & Hollander, E. (2002). *Anxiety disorders comorbid with depression: Social anxiety disorder, post-traumatic stress disorder, generalized anxiety disorder and obsessive–compulsive disorder.* London: Martin Dunitz.

Striegel-Moore, R. H., & Franko, D. I. (2004). Body image issues among girls and women. In T. F. Cash & T. Pruzinsky (Eds.), *Body image: A handbook of theory, research, and clinical practice* (pp. 183–191). New York: Guilford Press.

Tantleff-Dunn, S., & Gokee, J. I. (2004). Interpersonal influences on body image development. In T. F. Cash & T. Pruzinsky (Eds.), *Body image: A handbook of theory, research, and clinical practice* (pp. 108–116). New York: Guilford Press.

Vandereycken, W., & van Deth, R. (1994). *From fasting saints to anorexic girls: The history of self-starvation.* New York: New York University Press.

Werner, H. D. (1979). Cognitive theory. In F. J. Turner (Ed.), *Social work treatment: Interlocking theoretical approaches* (2nd ed., pp. 243–272). New York: Free Press.

Wolf, N. (1991). *The beauty myth.* New York: Anchor Books.

Additional Resources

Bakalar, N. (2007, December 11). Anorexia may be tied to hormones in womb. *New York Times.* Retrieved from http://www.nytimes.com/2007/12/11/health/research/11insi.html

Beck, A. T., & Rush, A. J. (1989). Cognitive therapy. In H. I. Kaplan & B. J. Sadock, B. J. (Eds.) *Comprehensive textbook of psychiatry* (5th ed., Vol. 2), pp. 1541–1550. Baltimore: Williams & Wilkins.

Calogero, W. R., & Davis, W. N. (2003, Summer). Self-objectification, body shame, media influence and eating disorders. *Perspectives: A Professional Journal of the Renfrew Center Foundation, 8,* 9–11.

Carvajal, D., (2008, April 16.) French bill takes chic out of being too thin. *New York Times,* p. A6.

Cash, T. F., & Pruzinsky, T. (Eds.) (2004). *Body image: A handbook of theory, reseach, and clinical practice.* New York: Guilford Press.

Chawla, S. (2000, November 24). Author deflects media blame for anorexia. *Washington Times,* p. 2.

DeRosis, H. A. (1979). *Women and anxiety: A step-by-step program to overcome your anxieties.* New York: Dellacorte Press.

Gans, H. (1966). Tradition and change in Italo-American family structure. In B. E. Segal (Ed.), *Racial and ethnic relations: Selected readings* (pp. 92–96). New York: Thomas Y. Crowell.

Goodman, W. K., Rudorfer, M. V., & Maser, J. D. (Eds.). (2000). *Obsessive–compulsive disorder: Contemporary issues in treatment.* Mahwah, NJ: Lawrence Erlbaum Associates.

Greenson, R. R. (1967). *The technique and practice of psychoanalysis* (Vol. 1). New York: International University Press.

Hamilton, G. (1951). *Theory and practice of social case work* (2nd ed., rev.). New York: Columbia University Press. (Original work published 1940)

Hearn, G. (1979). General systems theory and social work. In J. Turner (Ed.), *Social work treatment: Interlocking theoretical approaches* (2nd ed., pp. 333–360). New York: Free Press.

Herbert, J. D., Neeren, A. M., Lowe, M. R. (2007, Winter). Clinical intuition and scientific evidence: What is their role in treating eating disorders? *Perspectives: A Professional Journal of the Renfrew Center Foundation, 12,* 15–17.

Hollander, E. (2006). Obsessive–compulsive disorder. *Psychiatric Annals, 36,* 446–449.

Kirschenbaum, H., & Henderson, V. L. (Eds.). (1989) *The Carl Rogers reader.* Boston: Houghton Mifflin.

Kolata, G. (2007, November 11). Chubby gets a second look. *New York Times,* p. 4.

Malson, H. (1998). *The thin woman: Feminism, post-structuralism and the social psychology of anorexia nervosa.* New York: Routledge.

McKinley, N. M. (2004). Feminist perspective and objectified body consciousness. In T. F. Cash & T. Pruzinsky (Eds.), *Body image: A handbook of theory, research, and clinical practice* (pp. 55–64). New York: Guilford Press.

Minuchin, S., Rosman, B. L., & Baker, L. (1978). *Psychosomatic families: Anorexia nervosa in context.* Cambridge, MA: Harvard University Press.

Phillips, L. (1969). A social view of psychopathology. In P. London & D. Rosenhan (Eds.), *Foundations of abnormal psychology.* New York: Holt, Rinehart and Winston.

Pike, K. M., Devlin, M. J., & Loeb, K. L. (2004). Cognitive–behavioral therapy in the treatment of anorexia nervosa, bulimia nervosa, and binge eating disorder. In J. K. Thompson (Ed.), *Handbook of eating disorders and obesity* (pp. 130–163). Hoboken, NJ: John Wiley & Sons.

Pollack, M. H, Otto, M. W., & Rosenbaum, J. F. (Eds.). (1996). *Challenges in clinical practice: Pharmacologic and psychosocial strategies.* New York: Guilford Press.

Redlak, A. S., LeDay, R., & Boulter, C. (2007, Summer). The phase flow approach: An integrated recovery model. *Perspectives: A Professional Journal of the Renfrew Center Foundation, 12,* 9–11.

Roberts, R. W., & Nee, R. H. (Eds.). (1970). *Theories of social casework.* Chicago: University of Chicago Press.

Sinaikin, P. M., & Sachs, J. (1994). *Fat madness: How to stop the diet cycle and achieve permanent well-being.* New York: Berkley Books.

Smolak,L., & Murnen, S. K. (2004). A feminist approach to eating disorders. In J. K. Thompson (Ed.), *Handbook of eating disorders and obesity* (pp. 590–605). Hoboken, NJ: John Wiley & Sons.

Thompson, J. K. (Ed.). (2004). *Handbook of eating disorders and obesity.* Hoboken, NJ: John Wiley & Sons.

Turner, F. J. (Ed.). (1979). *Social work treatment: Interlocking theoretical approaches* (2nd ed.). New York: Free Press.

Wolf, N. (1993). *Fire with fire.* New York: Random House.

Index